From Shadows to Light

A Whole Human Approach to Mental Health

Compiled by Olivia Kachman

Published by Get You Visible

http://www.getyouvisible.com/

Print ISBN: 978-1-989848-06-7

eBook ISBN: 978-1-989848-07-4

Acknowledgments

Our families:

For being a source of support and love and/or for being a catalyst for change. Our lives have been shaped by your example, and it has motivated us to be the adults we are today.

Our ancestors:

For supporting our collective healing of any family trauma and/or mental health issues in our lineages, for all our Relations.

Our partners and friends:

For all those who have sat with us through the darkness, held our hands, listened without judgment, advocated for our recovery, and allowed us to borrow your strength and faith that "this too shall pass." Thank you for seeing our light when we could not and loving us no matter what.

Our health care team:

For helping us to navigate our diagnoses, supporting us through crises, listening with compassion, and believing in us when we did not believe in ourselves. Whether you are a mental health therapist, counsellor, social worker, medical doctor, psychologist, psychiatrist, naturopath, coach, mentor, holistic practitioner, spiritual guide, nutritionist, or fitness trainer - we honor your part in helping us rediscover our wellness.

Our publishing team:

For the leadership of CEO Heather Andrews of Get You Visible, support calls from Get You Visible business manager, Carrie-Ann Baron keeping everyone on track, the design skills of Lorraine Shulba, and the plethora of compassionate editors who have walked us through the process. We honor your guidance through difficult subject matter as you helped us to tell our stories.

Our fellow co-authors:

For sharing vulnerably, lifting each other up on hard days, and linking arms with courage knowing that we are stronger when we come together to make a difference.

Our compiler and contributing author, Olivia Kachman:

For not giving up on your life or this project despite being hospitalized for depression, anxiety, and acute suicidal ideation during the creation of this book.

Our readers:

For your own courage in ending the stigma around mental health. Thank you for supporting us by purchasing the book, recommending it to others, and contacting us personally if you were moved by our stories.

Table of Contents

Dancing in the Shadows: A Healer's Perspective on Mental Health Crisis

Conclusion

Afterword

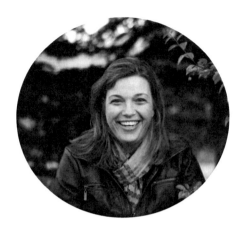

Foreword

By Rev. Carrie-Ann Baron

In your hands, you hold a collection of true stories that, when shared, can bring connection, inspiration and, most importantly, peer support to your mental health journey. Peer support is so important because it serves as an antidote to feelings of being alone and isolated - often the hardest part of managing mental health challenges.

In this compilation you will find a group of individuals who have been where you are and who are ready to connect and share their resources and tools for healing. Consider this reading a powerful first step toward connecting to a support system that takes a whole human approach to mental health.

Working with a support system that acknowledges you as a whole human (mind, brain, body and spirit) is a key component in moving from the shadows of mental health struggles into the light of health and positivity. The multi-disciplinary authors of this book courageously share their mental health stories, not through the limited lens of illness versus health, but rather from a holistic and compassionate perspective of recovery. These authors have chosen to share their recovery stories to offer you a feeling of inspired possibility.

As a trained peer support specialist and spiritual counsellor, I see this book as a valuable resource for anyone facing fear and doubt, wondering if life will ever get better. This book will help my clients, and so many others, explore a variety of therapeutic alternatives that could prevent a spiral deeper into the shadows and promote a deeper understanding of the power of vulnerability and connection in human betterment.

As someone who has lived her own experience with mental health, I see this book as a beacon of light. If I had the fortune to find this book while in the depths of my own shadows, I know it would have reassured me. It would have offered that it was okay to not be okay, that I was not alone in these thoughts and feelings and, finally, that asking for help would be a key component in bringing hope into my life. The authors acknowledge that the shadows are real and that, while the journey has been hard, moving from the shadows to light has been an important and meaningful process.

I first met Olivia at a Your Holistic Earth event several years ago where I was offering support to spiritual business owners in aligning their business and spiritual needs. Later, I began working with Heather Andrews, offering my assistance and support in building her publishing business. After a few short years, I found myself working with Heather and Olivia to bring Olivia's idea for this compilation to life. As the project moved forward, I was asked to offer my peer support services to the contributing authors of this book. It has been an honor to support Olivia and the authors in this capacity, and these stories have further validated the importance of peer support in healing, bringing the process full circle.

Before you turn the page and begin this journey, I invite you to close your eyes, take a deep breath and imagine that you are about to enter a very comforting and safe room. In this room is a circle of chairs, filled with kind faces welcoming you. The authors in this book are sitting around you, ready to share their stories, journeys, and learnings, all in a positive and empowering way. They are here to be with you and to support you exactly where you are at. Imagine yourself in this room, and with an open mind and a hopeful heart, turn the page and let the light in.

With love,
Rev. Carrie-Ann Baron

Ordained by The Canadian International Metaphysical Ministry

www.whitelightmetaphysical.com
https://www.facebook.com/whitelightmetaphysical
office@whitelightmetaphysical.com

Introduction

If you have experienced challenges with your mental health, you are an Initiate. You are a member of a select group of people with a common experience: you have felt the sting of undeserved stigma and navigated a broken health care system that has only limited resources to support your wellness and full recovery. Coping with compromised mental health can make you feel so alone, especially if your immediate family, friends, or colleagues have no clue what you are going through. Peer support is truly a lifesaver.

Whether you are an Initiate in search of inspiration, a caregiver looking for options to better support someone with mental health issues, or a health care professional open to learning about alternative approaches to mental health recovery, we welcome you to these pages wholeheartedly.

No matter what your personal experience of mental health or the recovery process has been, supporting those fumbling in the dark is often how you pay it forward as an Initiate. As an Initiate, you are the one who shows up and meets fellow travellers in the darkness with true empathy. You hold their hands and remind them to breathe through the cascade of tears and fears. You give validation, not unsolicited advice, or judgment. You provide living proof that this too shall pass, and that it is possible to feel better again.

What is rare is to find Initiates with in-depth lived experience and recovery perspectives among medical health care professionals.

The inspiration for *From Shadows to Light: A Whole Human Approach to Mental Health* was to provide important alternative resources to those who have struggled to find the support they need in the current health care system from those who have lived through mental health challenges and are providing services now that helped them get well.

All the co-authors wanted to give hope to others by telling their personal stories and speaking out as advocates for a better approach to mental health. It is not surprising that each of the co-authors lives in one of the most underfunded provinces for mental health initiatives: Alberta, Canada. Many of the Initiates who are co-authors in this compilation own wellness-based businesses, are professional speakers, and are making a difference in their workplaces and communities: they all are "being the change they wish to see" in the realm of a whole human approach to mental health.

Each of the eleven contributors brings a fresh perspective to mental health recovery:

- Dr. Christina Bjorndal and Katrina Breau are authorities on the role of nutrition in optimizing brain health and mental well-being.

- Ruthann Weeks shares her expertise in addressing systemic change by advocating for psychological safety in the workplace.

- Lisa and Mike Adams discuss their journey as a military family dealing with the consequences of PTSD.

- Vireo Karvonen and Cindy Klamn-Conway articulate their experiences overcoming shame and reclaiming their self-esteem.

- Marilyn Brighteyes powerfully reveals the devastating effects of intergenerational trauma from the Residential school genocide in Canada.

- Kimmy Krochak challenges the cultural norm that suggests that men deny their vulnerable emotions.

- Cinnamon Cranston and Olivia Kachman reveal the importance of body-based somatic healing, energy healing, and an emotional-spiritual approach to trauma recovery.

Each co-author is dancing between the shadows and the light. For some, the darkness remains ever-present, while for others, working within the "wounded healer" archetype is part of their growth and healing. Many have been thriving in their lives after years of serious issues but know they must be vigilant to prevent a relapse. We are all another reflection of you. By no means are we offering medical advice, rather, this book invites you to explore innovative themes and ideas as part of your own wellness recovery action plan.

It is our collective hope that our words will especially encourage other Initiates to not feel so alone and let them know that it is okay to not be okay! We are being brave, so you can be brave with us. Let us all challenge the stigma surrounding mental health together and question the current system that falls short of a whole human approach to health care that is accessible, affordable, and life-affirming for everyone.

If any of these stories, or parts thereof, trigger a negative emotional or psychological response for you, please do not hesitate to reach out for support immediately- to a friend, therapist, a crisis line or the authors in this book on Facebook @fromshadowstolightbook.

You never need to deal with your mental health alone.

Olivia Kachman

Dr. Christina Bjorndal

Dr. Christina Bjorndal, ND, is a naturopathic doctor who specializes in the treatment of depression, anxiety, bipolar disorders, and eating disorders. Having overcome many challenges herself, she has developed a highly effective approach to the treatment of 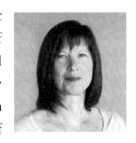 mental illness by addressing the needs of the whole person by taking into account physical, mental, emotional, and spiritual factors. Dr. Chris is a recognized authority in the naturopathic treatment of mental illness. A gifted writer and speaker, she has been invited to share her wellness philosophy on the Jenny McCarthy show and several docuseries, as well as at International Bipolar Foundation events and a variety of health summits. Her book *Beyond the Label* is a comprehensive guide to naturopathic mental health.

https://drchristinabjorndal.com/
https://www.facebook.com/drchrisbjorndal/
https://www.instagram.com/drchrisbjorndal/

Beyond the Label

By Dr. Christina Bjorndal

T hey say that growth happens through great struggle, and looking back, I can wholeheartedly confirm this has been true in my own life, and in the lives of my patients.

I am a naturopathic doctor committed to helping patients regain control of their mental health. It is a privilege to help people move past their labels and grow from their struggles. You see, I am also someone who has had to work through my own mental health challenges and overcome mental health labels.

My challenges were many: depression, suicide attempts, bipolar disorder type 1, bulimia, and anxiety. I've been there. I get it. In fact, if I add up all the times that I have been hospitalized, I have spent approximately one year of my life in a psychiatric ward. I weathered these labels and diagnoses for years, until I found natural integrative medicine and regained my mental health. Now, I guide others to do the same using a physical, mental, emotional, and spiritual approach to wellness.

***

While I was doing my undergraduate degree at the University of British Columbia in the late 1980s, I experienced a perfect storm. Under an intense amount of stress, I shouldered unrealistically high expectations of myself, and intense feelings of unworthiness that stemmed from being adopted. Subconsciously, I felt unwanted and afraid of rejection. I thought my self-worth was tied to my outward achievements, so I strove to compensate for my inner shame and fear with external accolades. Under all this stress, I thought that the only way "out" was to be the best. I pushed myself harder and harder. As my stress mounted, my survival and coping mechanisms were triggered.

Despite all my "success," my inner shame grew. When my achievements could no longer ease my feelings of stress and unworthiness, I resorted to bingeing and purging. Food and sugar became my primary means of dealing with stress, and I resorted to bulimia to avoid the consequences of my actions.

I had intense, paralyzing anxiety, driven by the feeling and belief that every decision I made had to be the *right* decision, as I was fearful of failure.

Eventually, I could not keep up and I fell into a suicidal depression. It did not go unnoticed by my family, friends, and coaches: I skipped practices, missed important deadlines, and was absent at social events. The worst part was dealing with the worsening thoughts of unworthiness that constantly plagued me.

One friend stepped in and made an appointment for me at the university student health clinic. This was the beginning of a long rollercoaster ride to recovery: a journey full of extreme highs and lows.

I was diagnosed with major depression and generalized anxiety. I was prescribed anti-depressants which I took faithfully without really understanding the treatment. I had grown up with the mentality that "the doctor knows best."

A few months later, I found myself in a state I had never experienced before. I was having sleepless nights, suddenly feeling absolutely euphoric, experiencing rapid speech and grandiose thoughts, all while acting extremely enthusiastic about everything. That lasted for a few days, until I unexpectedly spun into a full-blown delusional, psychotic manic episode. My physical and mental strength in a delusional state had me so wound up that it took six people to wrestle me into a straitjacket. I was taken to the hospital in an ambulance, where I was injected with a powerful anti-psychotic and left in a rubber room until I calmed down.

After that, I was moved to the psychiatric ward. The hospital psychiatrist diagnosed me with bipolar disorder type 1, a condition that typically presents with long stretches of depression marked by periodic swings to the opposite extreme state of mania, which was exactly what I had just experienced. Some people diagnosed with unipolar depression, can be triggered by anti-depressant medication and end up experiencing their first manic episode. This is what had happened to me. When I was discharged from the hospital, I was prescribed a new medication: lithium carbonate.

I somehow made it through the rest of university, despite being hospitalized again for my mental health during my senior year. I ended up attending my classes on a day pass from the hospital. I was nominated as the valedictorian of my graduating class that year and my parents were extremely proud of me. I, on the other hand, didn't think anything of this accomplishment. I was still stuck in the stigma and shame of my mental illness; of having experienced psychosis. I struggled with depression, anxiety, and bulimia. I wondered how I would move forward in life with these labels attached to me.

At first, the labels associated with my diagnoses were a relief; they provided an explanation for the symptoms that I was experiencing. They gave me something to point to that explained why I felt the way I did. I had an illness; it was not my fault. The only treatment option I was offered was pharmaceutical medication.

At the time, no one was talking about mental health in the media. Campaigns like Bell's 'Let's Talk Day' or Mental Health Awareness week didn't exist. Mental health was clouded in stigma and shame, and there was no public conversation about how to cope or support each other. I felt isolated, ashamed, and alone. So, instead of accepting my diagnoses, I pushed forward wearing the mask that everything was okay on the outside, when in reality, I was dying of shame on the inside. When I graduated from UBC, I went on to accept a high-stress job in the highly competitive field of commercial banking.

For the next decade, I pressed on, still wearing my "super-achiever" mask and burying not only my shame at not being good enough but also the belief that I had a diagnosis to hide. When I started working in the corporate world, my psychiatrist recommended that I not disclose my mental health history to my employer. This left me feeling as though having bipolar disorder type 1 was something to hide; that there was something inherently wrong with me.

I continued to struggle for the next few years, mostly with anxiety and depression. I learned to cope by driving my feelings deep below the surface. All these factors came to a head in 1994, when I was under immense pressure in a new position at the bank. I quickly found myself in a deeper depression than ever before. I floundered and felt isolated from the demands of my work. In addition to the mood stabilizing medication that I was already taking, my psychiatrist added an anti-depressant to my protocol in an attempt to lift the depression. While I wasn't comfortable with this poly-pharmacy approach, I took the medication as prescribed. After six months of struggling in my new role, and despite taking more medication, I attempted suicide on June 9, 1994[1].

I was not successful, but I ended up in a coma with kidney failure. When I regained consciousness, I was told I would need a kidney transplant. While I was recovering in the ICU, a friend gifted me *A Return to Love* by Marianne Williamson, a book that changed the course of my life. It helped me to take responsibility for my mental health and general well-being. I realized that being at war with myself was not serving me, so I began a spiritual quest to learn how to love and accept myself. It was then that I started to look for another way to manage my health and navigate the mental health labels that I had been given. Miraculously, my kidneys made a full recovery after receiving dialysis for several weeks.

***

After attending a Mental Health Regained Public Forum in 1999, I became a patient of Dr. Abram Hoffer, an orthomolecular psychiatrist, who prescribed nutritional treatments for psychiatric

---

[1] Suicidal ideation, thoughts, and behavior have long been linked to antidepressant usage. Selective serotonin reuptake inhibitors (SSRIs) including Zoloft are believed to increase suicidality risks. If you are depressed and reading this, please reach out for help by calling a loved one, a suicide hotline in your area, or 911 in North America.

conditions. I slowly regained my mental health through nutrition, natural supplements, and lifestyle changes, and I learned to love myself as I am, regardless of my achievements. By October 2000, I had experienced my first depression and anxiety-free year in 13 years.

I began the process of inquiry into what I really wanted to do with my life and finally mustered up the courage to resign from my corporate job. After sitting with the question, "If money didn't matter, what would I be doing?" The answer revealed itself in a tiny whisper: *Become a naturopathic doctor and help people heal from their mental health struggles using natural therapies and orthomolecular medicine, as you have been helped.*

I returned to high school at the age of thirty-three in order to get into the Faculty of Science at the University of British Columbia (UBC). Once at UBC, I took the pre-medical science courses required to get into the four-year naturopathic medicine program at the Canadian College of Naturopathic Medicine. It was difficult to reinvent myself at that stage of my life and I am grateful that I wasn't accountable to anyone else. I was free to start my life over again. Once at naturopathic medical school, I learned how to use nutrition and other modalities to address mental health concerns.

Since then, my journey has taken me across great distances of learning and growth. It's not as simple as saying that I have recovered my health and now help others from a place of "being healed." Living life while in recovery is an ongoing dance of self-care, self-acceptance, and humility. Self-love is a constant lesson: one that I am grateful to have the opportunity to learn over and over again, as it helps me guide others in learning it as well. I believe it is this vulnerability and honesty that leave me truly open and available to those that seek my help.

***

I chose to become a naturopathic doctor because I believe in the overarching model of how naturopathic medicine is delivered. Naturopathic medicine delivers natural treatments through nutrition and natural supplements, as well as therapies such as acupuncture, hydrotherapy, homeopathy, botanical medicine, and lifestyle counselling. The care is provided using a very important and unique approach: to find and treat the root cause of one's health concern. Questions to guide the inquiry include: When did it start? Where did the disease begin? What happened to the individual for mental illness to manifest in the first place?

My personal story did not start with the depressive symptoms I displayed at university, the bulimia, or my first manic episode. That was where doctors focused their questioning because those were the most intense manifestations of my mental state to date. No, my story started way back when I formed core beliefs about myself upon learning that I was adopted. I created a story in my head about what this said about me: that I wasn't worthy, wanted, or lovable. These beliefs were embedded in my subconscious mind and became the operating system that ran my life. To prove my worth and not get "sent back," I overcompensated by becoming an over-achiever. I was the top athlete in high school, the top student, and I won scholarships to attend university; however, I never learned how to manage stress and accept myself as I was. Instead, I sought meaning in prestige and awards, in being the best. My need to excel at everything all of the time led to anxiety and stress, which turned into an eating disorder, which

I then stuffed down into a depression that finally erupted into psychosis.

Genetics does play a role in mental illness, but so does one's personal history and psychology. Since I am adopted, I couldn't verify the truth of the gene theory of mental illness. Consequently, I continued to look for answers. I wanted to know what else makes a person likely to develop a condition or not. Epigenetics provided one possible answer. Studies show that brain development is not set in stone once a person reaches adulthood. It was once thought that genetics were stable and did not change, but we now know that although genes are the blueprint, they can be turned on or off, depending on the state of the cell (i.e. stressed, inflamed, calm, etc.) Take the brain, for example: epigenetics asserts that brain cells remain capable of growth, change, and modification throughout life; they are impacted by external factors such as stress. Our overall life experience (state of mind, exposures, food, toxins) serves to turn genes on or off, affecting our genetic expression and modifying our likelihood of developing a condition. Dr. Mehmet Oz explains, "genes load the gun, but lifestyle pulls the trigger."

This is why I decided to become a practitioner who offers an educated, evidence-based perspective that includes all levels of the experience of being alive. I want to contribute to a growing wave of holistic, integrative medicine that speaks to the spiritual aspect of health, one's emotions, past trauma, and core beliefs. I want to encourage the growth of the whole person, not just cover symptoms with medication. The holistic model moves beyond the body, into the mental, emotional, and even spiritual realms of human experience. This is a revolutionary model that has the power to change the methodology of human healing.

***

I have a vision for the future of medicine that is more about human evolution than it is about illness. I see a future where the body is treated as one with the mind and the soul. A future where conventional medicine embraces the holistic model and incorporates other modalities into mainstream treatment protocols. One where nutrition, psychology, and counselling are integrated into mental health treatments. I see a time when medicine will be sensitive to the deep fears a person may have about their illness, or being human, mortal, and in relationships. We will tap into people's intrinsic potential to be healthy. It all ties into how we treat our bodies and how we make decisions and form mental and physical habits in our daily lives.

Everyone knows we should eat healthy food, so why is it hard for us to choose the carrots over the cookies? As individuals, we are not just biology; we are a whole mass of nerves, thoughts, emotions, beliefs, energy, and cells that all tie in together with our worries about the past and future. Because we are so rarely present in the moment, making decisions about our health is more complicated than simply asking what is good or bad for us. Past events and experiences imprint on our subconscious mind, thereby influencing every decision we make in the present. For example, it took me over eight years to leave my corporate job. What would compel me to stay in a position that I had wanted to leave for so long? For me, it felt safer to endure a job that was draining my life energy, than risk rejection looking for another job. The subconscious belief guiding my decision was, "I am not wanted," which influenced how I operated in the world. Once I was able to bring conscious awareness to what was driving my behaviour, I was able to make a change. Even small decisions, like deciding what to have for lunch, are filtered through the thick lenses of all that we carry with us. If we want to heal people and help them build truly good, long-term habits, we must take a holistic approach; otherwise, all the "stuff of life" will continue to get in the way of our efforts.

It follows that it is extremely important to have a good, respectful working relationship with one's doctors. Being able to spend time with your health care providers and have them understand who you are and where you are coming from is integral to creating a sustainable, manageable, medically appropriate, long-term treatment plan. Being part of a community is even more conducive to healing, as there is a beneficial effect to working as a group. It is easier to make healthy life choices when you are surrounded by others with similar goals, guided by the same efforts.

The future of mental health care lies in understanding the root causes of mental health issues. Currently only 5.5% of the Canadian health care budget is spent on preventative medicine.[2] If we spent more money in education and early intervention, the massive costs of invasive and dramatic hospital and

---

[2] Canadian Institute for Health Information, National Health Expenditures Database:
https://apps.cihi.ca/mstrapp/asp/Main.aspx?Server=apmstrextprd_i&project=Quick%20St ats&uid=pce_pub_en&pwd=&evt=2048001&visualizationMode=0&documentID=9D0E83 BC4BACDADE9D4938B338C6B6D5&_ga=2.49592614.1456706886.1566520003-763161464.1566520003 & Hammerstein et al, 2016: https://www.ncbi.nlm.nih.gov/pmc/articles/PMC4695931/

pharmaceutical medicine would be reduced. Truly investing in prevention by spending 10% of the national budget would be an excellent way to reduce the incidence, suffering, and costs of illness. It is forward thinking to keep people healthy rather than treating them after they are ill. Why then are we not investing more in prevention? True illness prevention starts with healthy communities, healthy relationships, and healthy psyches. This is a daunting concept for a model of medicine that has traditionally only focused on the body.

***

An ideal holistic model of mental health care would involve several layers, or realms, of preventative intervention, starting at the foundation: with children. Children should be taught models of self-care from a very young age, starting with self-love, rather than shame or blame. However, in order for children to learn effectively, parents must also have been taught these skills.

Our school system needs to change to value emotional intelligence and qualities like kindness and compassion, as much as it values reading, writing, and arithmetic. Learning institutions should actively encourage, prioritize, and facilitate healthy food choices, movement, and exercise.

In the corporate sector, businesses should foster work-life balance by creating new models for work schedules that allow for mental health flex days and appropriate leave allowances, rather than the current stringent system of limited sick days and minor support for long-term or stress leave.

In the current political climate, naturopathic medicine is not funded by the government, and many people who truly need the care of a naturopathic doctor do not have access. Mental health therapy and counselling should be financially accessible and completely normalized as a healthy thing to do. There should be no stigma around seeing a counsellor or getting guidance from a professional for your mental health. Governments should support all of these initiatives by lowering the barriers to care by funding preventative and community programs that provide the less fortunate with access to health-promoting foods, environments, and services.

In short, capitalism and profiteering need to be kicked out of the ring; health promotion should be guided by long-term strategies created with the health of the population as the number one priority. Once a larger percentage of the federal health care budgets are focused on healthy lifestyle habits in children and in the workplace, we will be on our way to an effective, sustainable and preventative mental health care system.

How can we, as individuals, contribute to the creation of a better health care system in the future? We can all be fierce advocates for mental health in our own way. The first step is to fight the stigma surrounding mental health, which begins by simply talking about it, by being open and honest about our own struggles, and those of the people that we support. Individuals need to face, accept, and admit that mental health is a real concern for many of us, and that there is no shame in that.

Additionally, we need to encourage open-minded discussions about the various philosophies of treating mental illness. Committing to a single model slows growth and contributes to stagnation. We need to invite open conversations and be more accepting of alternative medicine. The medical community needs to understand that, as professionals, we need to work together as a team to support the best interests of patients. We also need to be realistic about the risks and benefits of all treatments, including the very real risks of pharmaceutical treatment. Essentially it is not about incorporating only conventional medicine or alternative medicine but utilizing both systems together in an integrative fashion. We also need to integrate different systems of medicine, and support those who are at the forefront of integrative medicine, like naturopathic doctors, osteopaths, chiropractors and acupuncturists. The goal is not to replace any one form of medicine, but to use each tool according to its strengths, with a minimum amount of invasive intervention.

Mental health is not just about the illness, it is about the whole person. And, likewise, reforming mental health care is not just about deciding what medicines to administer; it is about how our entire culture views and treats mental health. If internal healing begins with self-acceptance, self-compassion, and self-love, then treating the national mental health epidemic will begin with cultural acceptance, reduction of shame, and the cultivation of love.

Personal Insights: From Shadows to Light

- NOURISH: Eating a diet that did not properly nourish my body contributed to years of depression. I had to learn to give my body the proper building blocks to even have a chance to be healthy.
- CALM: Stress is often the root cause of many mental and physical issues. It causes so many issues that stress management must be a part of any healing journey.

- MOVE: Regular exercise has been shown to be as effective as antidepressants for mild-to-moderate depression.[3] You can do it!
- REST: Sleep loss raises stress hormones (cortisol) and disrupts the balance of additional hormones that affect energy and digestion. Protecting sleep is a foundational way to promote mental well-being.
- REFLECT: My healing did not begin in earnest until it came from a place of self-acceptance, self-compassion and self-love. I had to learn to let go of self-blame, shame, and fear.
- ENGAGE: True recovery happens when you feel included and empowered in your care. This is especially true for preventative medicine, because you must be an active participant engaged in making healthy lifestyle and behavioral choices.
- BE PATIENT: Healing may never be "complete," rather, it is a circle of continuous growth and learning. A part of your healing journey must also be forgiving yourself if you have setbacks.
- HELP: You can be helpful to others even when you are on your own healing journey. Don't think you have to be "all fixed" before you help others.

---

[3] (source: https://www.health.harvard.edu/mind-and-mood/exercise-is-an-all-natural-treatment-to-fight-depression)

Lisa and Mike Adams

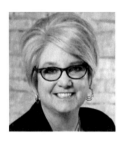

Lisa Adams is a Life Coach, fitness trainer, and professional speaker. Lisa has been a part of the military family for over 20 years. She brings a unique approach to dealing with trauma that stems from her marriage to a military member who was injured and diagnosed with PTSD in 2006. Lisa has experience working as an Education Assistant supporting students with trauma issues, special needs and learning disabilities. She has been a volunteer with the Peer Support Program with Operational Stress Injury Social Support (OSISS) for the past 3 years.

Lisa has multiple diplomas in Professional PTSD Counselling, Fitness and Nutrition, Personal Training, as well as certifications in Cognitive Behaviour Techniques, Empowerment Life Coaching, Reiki Master, and Advanced Angel Empowerment Practitioner. Lisa is continually updating her trauma training. Her mission is to "Educate and empower, one person at a time."

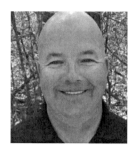 **Michael Adams** is currently a serving member in the Canadian Armed Forces. Michael's career started over 23 years ago as a member of Princess Patricia's Canadian Light Infantry. He is currently a Land Communication and Information System Technician. He has had multiple deployments both domestic and international.

www.heart.support
www.facebook.com/reducingtrauma
lisa@heart.support

From Battlefield to Home

By Lisa and Mike Adams

Too often the stigma and shame associated with Post Traumatic Stress Disorder (PTSD) forces people into the shadows and prevents them from seeking the help they need. They feel alone, isolated, and hopeless.

After years of working through our own demons, Mike and I have learned that suffering in silence is not the answer. Nothing is ever solved by staying in the shadows. Recovery lies in education, communication, sharing, and bringing the struggle into the light.

If you suffer from the effects of trauma and PTSD, we want you to know that you are not alone and that you have nothing to be ashamed of. We are living proof that there is hope and that there is a way out of the darkness.

This is our story.

Mike

Sweat, why am I sweating so much? Fuck, I hate them, I hate them all. Why did it have to be my boys, my soldiers, my friends and not me, that had to die? They were so young and had a full life to live. My God, that smell! What is that horrible, rancid odor? Why is it so hot? I am at home, in Canada, am I not? Where am I? Where is my gun? Is this my day, the day that I die? Being shaken awake only to realize that I am in the safety of my own bed and lying in a pool of my own sweat.

I'm embarrassed because I am supposed to be the strong one in my household; I am the protector. I'm thinking, *what is wrong with me? I am not broken*. Yeah, I got hurt and had to be sent out of the operational area for surgery, but I wasn't going to die. Did my wife shake me awake because I was screaming out loud in my sleep, or were my screams just in my head? But when I woke up, my wife Lisa was still fast asleep.

Afghanistan smelled like death in every direction. That and the constant smell of shit; all day, every day. The smells let us know we were still here in Afghanistan. Our sixteen-man tent on a slab of concrete was our home for a long time. No AC. It was so hot in the desert, we didn't need any heaters, but we really could've used some AC, or working AC. Our first night on the ground was also our first exposure to a rocket attack; seven rockets were launched into the camp. Per standing orders, drills were supposed to be conducted for the safety of all people staying within the confines of the camp. We conducted those drills only once by the book, and what we found is that there were not enough concrete bunkers for all of the members in the camp. So, from that night forward, we stayed where we hoped the next rocket launched into the camp by the Taliban wouldn't find us; ninety-nine percent of the time, that was just in our beds.

The Taliban were relentless on the days they attacked. They changed their attack strategies each time to keep us confused, just as we did to them. They found that roadside bombs were an effective means to kill, maim, or injure Canadian and Allied troops. The first week I was there, we had to conduct a ramp ceremony for a group of Americans that had been attacked during a convoy. The death did not bother me, but what I couldn't get out of my head was a young American soldier who'd lost half his face. His jaw was hanging off; the bandages were barely keeping it in place. He was slumped over from injury but was determined to carry the casket of his fallen brother in arms. It was at that moment that I developed true hatred for the Taliban.

Convoys were an everyday occurrence while in theatre (the place of deployment) and the risk was high for engagement with the Taliban, or with villagers whom the Taliban had paid or promised to protect if they attacked us. Now that IEDs (roadside bombs) were the newest and biggest threat to our safety, we stayed in a constantly vigilant state, knowing full well that complacency would kill us or others. Knowledge was power and power was everything in this place. If you had power, you had control. I didn't have power by the rank and position I held, but what I did have, was knowledge. My job was Counter Roadside Bomb Specialist, equipping our convoys with the protective measures against IEDs.

Boom! There it was: an IED attack followed by a ground attack, right next to the Kandahar Airfield.

Looking back, it was quick; in the moment it seemed to last for hours. The insurgents were killed and there were many injured. I was on the phone with my wife when the loudspeaker rang out, "The following blood types must get to Charlie role immediately: O neg., O pos., AB neg." Even my wife heard the explosion and the call for help. I hung up and left her on the telephone not knowing what was going on, what was happening. I can't speak for her, but I am sure she was confused or scared.

When I was sent home with a physical injury in 2006, I didn't know that I was also mentally injured. My wife and I were in the so-called honeymoon phase of my post-operational tour, as well as our relationship. I was glad to be home- to spend time with my family; have intimate, physical contact with my wife- to enjoy all of the positive stuff you miss while deployed.

As this post-tour honeymoon phase wore off, I knew something wasn't right. I didn't know what was happening to me. I was angry. I was withdrawn. I was panicked to attend events with friends, go to the mall, or visit crowded places. I was continually watching people, having to know where their hands were (hand checking). I felt hatred for a whole culture of people (over there, nobody could be trusted as they were easily paid off to kill one of us). Sleep? What was sleep? I would get at most forty minutes of sleep in any given twenty-four-hour period. I stopped working out, stopped eating even half-way healthy. I didn't feel I belonged on this planet, didn't feel safe, even in my own house. I had no gun. Nothing in life mattered.

I was desperate and isolated. I had no self-worth and no sense of community. I had a couple of outbursts in my home; nothing physical, but there were angry words. Once I refocused, I saw the impact it was having on my family. I couldn't live with myself seeing them upset, scared, and intimidated by my presence. From that moment on, I decided to suffer in silence. My wife didn't know what was going on with me; I didn't know what was going on with me. PTSD was only a label at that time.

When our medical system finally caught up with me and they made me fill in my "return from tour documentation," I actually answered all of the questions truthfully. They sat me down with a CAF mental health professional almost immediately.

I was assigned a psychologist and went through direct exposure therapy. It was tough at first. I, like many others, didn't want to talk to someone who hadn't been there. How can you possibly know what I am going through if you weren't there? By the end of my therapy, I had a toolbox of mental actions I could use to get me through a triggered event.

For those of us living with PTSD, life is far from "normal." We push people away, we get used to losing relationships and friendships, we no longer enjoy our favorite pastimes, we feel irritated, we get mad easily, and we have a very hard time coping with any anniversary related to the cause of our PTSD.

Some people stare, others say, "What's wrong with him?" Some people call it "anger," some call it "triggered." Psychologists use "hyperarousal," "depression," or "anxiety," and other medical terms that we don't understand, to describe what is happening to us. They offer us a variety of different treatments like CPT (Cognitive Processing Therapy), CBT (Cognitive Behavioral Therapy), PET (Prolonged Exposure Therapy) and send us to the psychiatrist who prescribes Zoloft, Paxil, Prozac, SSRIs (antidepressants), Zopiclone, Prazosin, Effexor, marijuana, and the list goes on.

Call it brainwashed or forced mental pressures, but whatever you call it, the combination of our training and experience keeps us alive in theatre and makes it really hard to reintegrate into normal life when we come home. As soldiers, we are trained before we are sent to any peacekeeping, peace-making, or war environments. In 2006, I was training for war in Afghanistan, which involved a continuum of forever changing scenarios taken from lessons learned in previous deployments. When we train, we rely on repetition to ensure our drills are so second nature that we don't question our abilities when we go into combat. What we are not prepared for is the actual operational environment: heat, sandstorms, the smell of fecal matter all day long, and living in the middle of a shooting range knowing that someone is trying to kill us.

I had a relapse in 2015. This time that mental toolbox they gave me in 2007 couldn't pull me through my triggered state. I tried to end my life at least seven times over the next few months. When my youngest child almost caught me in the act, I realized that I couldn't do that to him. I couldn't make him live with finding his dad dead. Again, I sought help. This is when I started building a true and truthful relationship with my family, as there was nothing left to hide. Homework with, or in the presence of my wife, was part of my recovery process. Lisa was involved throughout, engaging with me, asking questions. They weren't always the right questions and not always at the right time, but my family's presence was necessary for me to heal.

Lisa

The morning was here. He would be leaving on his chalk (military flight) headed to Kandahar and a few hours later I would be flying back to Victoria. I didn't know what to expect that day, my emotions were all over the place. He was in his routine. He had deployed before, and he knew the drill. I was trying to keep my emotions under control, although it felt like I was losing a piece of my heart.

We got to the LTF (Learning Training Facility) where all the chalks would be leaving from. We walked in holding hands like we always did. The drill hall was huge and, as we walked in, we could see that some families and their soldiers were already there. Mike introduced me to some of them. Then we were asked to sit down because the CO was going to address the group.

When the CO was finished, it was time for all of the members to start their DAG process, which basically means that they finished their preparations by going from table to table collecting the last items they needed before boarding the bus that was to transport them to the airport. I can remember that one table contained cash and another the bolt to his weapon. I had no idea what a bolt was until he explained it to me.

I could feel my emotions welling up, but I wanted to keep it together, so I tried my hardest to keep my emotions under control. He looked at me and said, "Well, it's that time," and I knew exactly what that meant. He said, "I am going to walk you out to the car." He didn't want to say goodbye in front of everyone. We walked out holding hands and got to his friend Jason's car; that's when the floodgates opened. I couldn't hold them back anymore. Tears were streaming down my face and I was hugging him so tightly; I didn't want to let him go.

The following March, our friends asked if Mike and I wanted to do a double wedding when he came home on his HLTA (on leave). Before he left, I had made a bet with Mike that we would never get married, but to my surprise, when I brought it up on a call a few days later, he said yes! It was originally going to be just be the four of us getting married in Edmonton, but as it turned out, Mike and I ended up getting married in Victoria accompanied by 70 friends and family. We later attended the other couple's wedding in Edmonton.

We planned our wedding together via calls and MSN conversations. He sent me his tux info and I ordered it. He had no idea what it looked like. He flew home on Friday, April 7, 2006. I picked him up from the airport, and we went to pick up his tux. Twenty-four hours later we were married. I was now Mrs. Michael Brian Adams Jr. He didn't just make a commitment to me but also to my son Alexander. To mark the occasion, en route from Kandahar, he purchased our rings and a beautiful necklace and ladybug pendant for Alex in Dubai.

Our wedding was perfect. Our family and friends were there to celebrate that wonderful day with us. As Mike tells it, I was late, and I spat out my gum into my Dad's hand while walking down the aisle.

The next day, Mike's mom let me know that she was glad I was now his wife and that she wouldn't be the one who would get the "Phone Call" if something should happen to him while he was deployed, which really put things into perspective for me. By this time in 2006, a number of soldiers had already been killed.

During Mike's short leave, we also travelled to Edmonton to attend our friends' wedding and returned to Victoria to find a new family home.

It was then, when we had just moved into our new house, that I first saw what a PTSD episode looked like. I couldn't tell you what time it was, but one night a loud car alarm suddenly sounded from the driveway next door. As soon as it went off, my husband tucked and rolled out of bed onto the floor looking for his clothes. Not knowing what was happening, I laughed hysterically at him. He told me that in camp, when a rocket flies into camp and the siren goes off, they roll out of bed, get dressed, and go to the bunker. I was glad that he had shared this information with me, but I still didn't fully understand what was happening to him and wouldn't for some time after that.

Then it was time for my husband to head back to Afghanistan.

I think it was harder to watch him leave this time, as his wife. Somehow, being a spouse, made it harder knowing that even in camp he wasn't safe. Now, I worried even more than I ever had before.

June 2006 was the worst month of my life. I was on my computer at work sending emails, calling clients, and chatting on MSN, when Mike popped online. To be honest, I can't remember how the conversation even started but I clearly remember him saying, "So what do you think if I came home early?" My mind started swirling. I knew he wasn't joking and that something had happened. My reply was "What's going on; are you injured?" Or something to that effect. No sooner had I typed out those words than the phone on my desk rang. I had butterflies in my stomach. I answered and it was Mike.

He said that the doctor there had found a tumor on his testicle and that he was being sent home to see a specialist to find out if it was malignant or not. I felt like everything was happening in slow motion and I couldn't focus on anything else. I went to my supervisor and told him what was happening. He sent me home. On the way, I called my sister Nadine who works at a cancer clinic, and by the time Mike was back in Canada, he already had an appointment booked with the best urologist in Victoria.

The next few days were mostly a blur. Mike went to his doctor at the MIR, met with the urologist, and booked his surgery date. It was mid-July. After the procedure, it was a waiting game. We just had to sit tight until they could tell us if his tumor was malignant or not. Anyone who has gone through this process themselves or with a loved one, knows how stressful it is to live in that "what if" place, not knowing what the outcome will be. The mind plays out so many possible scenarios and outcomes. Little did I know that Mike would be okay, although, as a result of the surgery, we would have problems conceiving.

It was at that time that Mike went over to Mental Health to fill out the paperwork and answer questions about the effect of deployment on his mental status. He knew what the "right" answers were if he wanted to appear healthy and avoid jeopardizing his career. He also realized that he now had a new life with a wife and stepson. Giving the "correct" answers wouldn't help us as a family, so he did what many soldiers are afraid to do; he answered honestly. The unfortunate thing is that even now in 2019, military members still lie on their mental health forms because of the ongoing stigma associated with PTSD.

During the first few years of his diagnosis, Mike had many PTSD episodes. The diagnosis provided a label to describe his behavior, but that doesn't mean we understood was really going on with him. After a while, we just knew it could happen at any time. Some incidents stand out more than others.

That October 2006, we went to Edmonton on a family trip to visit our friends and meet our goddaughter. A few days before we were scheduled to go back to Victoria, we all decided to go to breakfast at an ABC restaurant. When we were finishing up our meal and the waitress was collecting the empty dishes, the utensils fell off a maple syrup covered plate. They landed right on Mike's arm and leg. He reacted by screaming and yelling profanities at her. I looked at him and said, "Leave your wallet and go outside for a smoke." In other words, *oh no, this will not go well if he stays here.* Mike got up and went outside, leaving our friends and their kids wondering what in the hell had just happened? Even though Mike didn't want anyone to know, I explained that he had been diagnosed with PTSD. I felt that I had to tell them because otherwise they would think he had just gone crazy. At least this way, they had a reason for it, even if they didn't really know what it was.

Later, in December, I was excited to be going to Mike's work Christmas party and meeting more of his work friends. I remember that we stopped by his boss's house first for drinks and then went on to the party for the Junior Ranks. Mike's friend, Chad, was home from the same deployment. They had been the first two to deploy to Afghanistan from Victoria, so there was a bond between them.

As with most other Christmas parties, there was plenty of alcohol flowing. The drinks kept coming and the testosterone kept building. Chad and one of Mike's subordinates were playing around and wrestling. Like our mothers always told us, it is all fun and games until it's not. The friendly wrestling escalated to something more aggressive. That's when my husband went from watching and laughing, to a full-on PTSD episode. It happened so fast.

It was as if the subordinate was a target in a war zone and Chad was being assaulted. I should mention that Chad was a very fit guy and the subordinate was a younger fella and not as strong. All Mike could see was a target and only the target. He locked on and was going to kill the subordinate with his bare hands. He ran over and jumped into the action, then a bunch of other guys started jumping on top of them.

In a split second the party went from having fun with friends to ten guys holding my husband back, preventing him from attacking that young man. Mike was yelling and saying that he was going to kill the kid, that there would be nothing left of him. What scared me the most was when I went up and stood eye to eye with him, trying to get his attention. I was saying "Mike, Mike look at me! Talk to me!" He looked right past me, still locked on to his target, still yelling. I was really scared. I had never seen anyone in that type of rage.

His sergeant intervened and told him that he would be charged if he didn't stop. Mike heard that, but his response wasn't to stop but to yell out his service number. The sergeant kept yelling at him and I finally yelled, "He has PTSD!" I was dumbfounded at the sergeant's response: "What's that?" Now more like a protective momma bear I went on the attack myself. "It's post-traumatic stress disorder, you asshole!" But, it still didn't seem to register with him.

By now the military police had been called and the Christmas party was over. Thank goodness one of our friends, another sergeant, managed to get Mike calm enough to sneak out the back way and into a car. By the time the police arrived, we were no longer there.

Even now, looking back, I can still see every last detail of that night because it was a traumatic experience for me.

We got through the rest of the winter unscathed and continued doing well until baseball season started up the following June. I can vividly remember one particular tournament playoff game when a guy on the other team started yelling and screaming at our team. At first, Mike just countered with some comments of his own, but then something the guy said triggered him and he went into a full-blown PTSD episode. He headed over to the other bench to "end his life." He was in a rage. This time, a couple of our friends- including the best man at our wedding- and I, were able to calm him down enough so he wouldn't hurt the guy and we could finish the ball game.

Earlier in May we had found out that we were going to be posted to Kingston, Ontario, and that we had a short window of time to see a fertility specialist before we moved. We had been trying, unsuccessfully, to get pregnant for almost a year. At the clinic, Dr. Hudson determined that because of Mike's injuries to his testicles, our best chance for conceiving would be to undergo fertility treatments.

It had been determined that Mike's injuries had been caused by the ionized and nonionized radiation coming from the new electronic counter measures (ECMs) that were being employed to prevent the explosion of roadside bombs and keep our military members safe. Mike was unaware of the dangers of the radiation coming from the equipment he was installing on the military vehicles.

We started with the injections on the day we first visited Kingston to find a new house in anticipation of our July posting.

I was about ten weeks pregnant with twins when we started our drive across Canada and was experiencing morning or all-day sickness. The drive wasn't the best and I couldn't wait to get to Kingston. I knew that when we got there, the doctors could check on the babies. I went in for my ultrasound with Mike beside me. The technician took her time and then left the room. She came back in followed by a colleague to consult with. Mike and I could see that there were two sacs and one baby, but what did we know? A few minutes later, the doctor told us that there was only one baby. He described what had happened as Vanishing Twin Syndrome. All we knew was that we had lost a baby.

The next day, I was still feeling emotional after the loss of the twin when the movers met us at our new Kingston home. I recall that it was a beautiful, sunny day. I was checking off the box numbers as they were being taken off the truck. The day was progressing, and the movers were getting careless and damaging our belongings. My husband was inside the house, directing the movers to the appropriate rooms.

At one point in the afternoon I overheard the younger guys sitting out front where I was. I clearly remember that one was saying that he was under house arrest and that he was glad that they hadn't damaged anything that day. I turned to him and said, "You dropped my dresser down the stairs, and you carried our washer into house by yourself and damaged that." I continued to list the items I knew had been damaged. He looked at me and called me, "a lying, fucking bitch." I was shocked and immediately got up out of my lawn chair. I went into the house to the living room where my husband and the truck driver were. I told them what had happened. The words were barely out of my mouth before my husband was chasing the young man down the road.

I was afraid of what might happen because I knew that Mike was emotional about the twin and very protective of me. I called the military police to ensure the event was documented. They came to the house and drafted a report. I also called the moving company and a supervisor soon arrived. When I got off the phone, my husband was back with the young man in tow. The mover was given an ultimatum: if he didn't apologize, he wouldn't be alive to worry about being under house arrest. The young man apologized. He then went over and sat down by the curb.

Those are only some of the episodes we experienced in the early days; there were others. Although we did learn to spot potential triggers, we were never really sure when the next incident would occur. That's the thing with PTSD, it's unpredictable.

We slowly came to terms with the loss of the twin and focused on getting ready to welcome our baby into the world. Mike was doing great and was in what is termed PTSD remission. He wasn't having episodes and things were going well for us.

That year, Alex was spending the Christmas holidays in Victoria, so Mike gave me a ticket to fly out on Boxing Day to see my son and spend time with my sister who was also pregnant. I flew back home to Kingston on December 30; we were planning a couple's night out for New Year's Eve. It would be our last chance before the baby came in February.

By the time I got home, I already wasn't feeling well. By New Year's Eve the next day, I was really feeling sick. But I knew that the tickets for the gala were expensive, so I went anyway. Boy, I definitely wasn't prepared to bring in the New Year the way we did.

It was after the meal, Mike was enjoying himself, mingling and having sociables. After all, this was going to be the last big party before our little one entered the world.

It was about 11:40 p.m., and my contractions were coming strong and often. I said to Mike, "I think it's time we go to the hospital." Our little monkey was coming, and nothing was going to stop him. He was born January 1, 2008, the first in Kingston, third in Ontario, and fifth in Canada to be born on that day. We were overjoyed that our little boy was finally here. But, Lochlynd Michael Clarence had arrived early. He was born by C-section and it was touch and go there for a while. Thankfully, after twenty-one days in the NICU, he was able to come home safe and sound.

Honestly, by then I hated being in Kingston, even though it was beautiful. With everything we had been through, I just didn't want to be there anymore. But, moving meant that in all likelihood Mike would again be deployed to Afghanistan or some other dangerous place. In Kingston, he was posted to the Signals School, which meant that he wasn't at risk. In the end, I couldn't take it anymore and I told him that I didn't care if he had to be deployed again, I didn't want to stay in Kingston. Still, we were stuck there for two years before we were finally posted back west; to Edmonton this time.

We arrived in Edmonton on August 1, 2009 and settled into the PMQ that has been our home for the past ten years. We've done well and we've been luckier than some because, even if PTSD has put our family through hell, we've also had joy and good times.

Life had been good since our move to Edmonton, but in June of 2013, Mike was redeployed to Afghanistan. Of course, I was concerned that he would be retraumatized and that all of the progress he had made, all of the work he had done in therapy, would go out the window.

He returned in December and, this time, he seemed to be doing really well. I would only notice little triggers when we were in crowds or at a friend's house and new people would show up. All the military guys, including Mike, would stand against the wall. They would check out the new people and where their hands were. Similarly, when we would go out to eat, Mike would have his back to the wall. He would know where the exits were, how many people were in the restaurant, and be hyper focused on all the activity around him. This became so normal that I started doing the same thing when I went out with my friends. That being said, by 2013, we seemed to be in a much better place than before.

Lochlynd had started Grade 1 while Mike was deployed overseas and Alex, Grade 10. There is an inside joke among military families that things wait for the member to deploy before going wrong, but this time was different for us. There were some issues while Mike was away, but the kids and I fared pretty well; better than usual. I was an EA at one of the schools and the kids were busy with summer, then hockey.

I had been looking forward to December 11, 2013. That was the day that Mike would be returning from his deployment.

We had decided not to tell the boys that Dad was coming home; we wanted to surprise them. We first went to Lochlynd's school where he was having his Christmas concert. Mike waited behind a gym curtain so Lochlynd wouldn't see him. As the song was coming to an end, Mike walked up the aisle. Lochlynd's eyes grew wide and he waved to his Dad. He knew he wasn't supposed to get off the stage, so he waited until he was told he could.

We headed to the high school with Lochlynd, to surprise Alex. When we entered his classroom, he had his nose in a book, pretending to read. His friend told him to look up. When he saw Mike, he jumped out of his seat and walked up to the front of the class to give him a huge hug. It was amazing to see how excited the boys were to have Dad home.

In the spring of 2014, we found out Mike was going to be posted to Red Deer. We decided as a family that the boys and I would stay in Edmonton because Alex was in high school. Mike would travel home weekly from Red Deer to make sure we had as much family time as possible. That was our routine until 2015. Little did we know what the next two years would bring.

It is at this time that we started to realize just how profound and persistent the effects of PTSD are on the injured individual and those close to them. Until 2015, we had treated PTSD mostly as Mike's problem; something he needed to work on. I was not as aware of how much it had directly affected me or the children. I did not realize that we were all suffering from PTSD; we had all been injured. We needed to heal, as individuals and as a family. That was a turning point for us: that is when the real healing began. We're not done yet. It is an ongoing process, but we understand so much more now.

It was also a difficult year for us. I had a serious work accident in September that left me with a traumatic brain injury. I was incapacitated for three months before WCB sent me to the head injury clinic. I worked with a therapist to help me heal physically and mentally. I was concerned about returning to work. And, in fact, the teacher I worked for as a teaching assistant didn't understand that I was doing the best I could and made my life very difficult.

That was also the year that the wife of one of Mike's subordinates was having mental health issues and attempted suicide a number of times. Her situation would seriously impact our lives. One of those times, Mike was on the phone with his subordinate while she was trying to cut herself. We called the EMS and the police and got her some help. She was admitted to the psych hospital to be monitored.

The next day, Mike went over to their house. I didn't know it then, but the heat in the house and the smell of blood put him right back in Afghanistan. That's when he started coming out of remission. Then, he was triggered again when he visited her at the hospital. None of us expected that this incident would send him for another ride on the PTSD rollercoaster but, eventually, he came to me and told me that he needed to go check in with Mental Health.

Mike played down the seriousness of his relapse, but I noticed that he wasn't sleeping much, if at all.

This time, we did things a bit differently: we decided to treat the PTSD as a family issue. When Mike went back to seek mental health support, so did our whole family. Alex saw a social worker on base, Lochlynd visited a child psychologist, I sought help through Alberta Mental Health, and Mike saw his own therapist. Lochylnd also participated in a program called iSTEP, a program that helps kids living with a member who has PTSD or OSI (Operational Stress Injury). It provides them with tools and techniques to help them cope.

Part of our process was that we would check in after our appointments to see how we were all doing. One day, after one of my sessions, I came home and was trying to tell Mike something that I had unsuccessfully tried to communicate before. It hadn't come out right the first time. That's when I got his gut punching response: "Since we are being honest, I need to tell you that I have flirted with suicide thirteen times." I could feel my jaw opening in shock. I think that I said, "You can't die on me."

I didn't ask a lot of questions, but I recall conversations about how close he really was to leaving this world. I felt so guilty that I hadn't recognized how bad things had gotten for him. I felt that I had failed him as a wife. It also really brought home how serious our situation was and, how if someone really wanted to end their life, they could just go and do it without anyone seeing the signs.

I was very grateful to have my OSISS Peer Support community to help me work through and process what was happening. It was encouraging to speak to other spouses who also had experience with PTSD at home.

As Mike got better, my mental health declined. I disassociated from people and really didn't leave my house anymore. I was doing the work because I wanted us to be successful on our mental health journey, but conventional therapy wasn't really helping me. Then I had an opportunity to try equine therapy and everything changed. I improved more in a few weeks than I had in two years. I began to understand that I had trouble sharing my emotions and that's when I really started opening up about some of my own trauma. My healing process had finally begun for real.

It is now 2019 and, compared to when I first met him, Mike is a 3.0 version of himself. He has learned that self-care, working out, golfing, playing ball, and spending time with family helps him in his recovery.

For my part, after being a part of the OSISS community for a year, I became a Peer Support Volunteer. I now help share information about PTSD and support other families. I support them and help them understand the triggers, behaviors, and symptoms of PTSD. I also share our family's story. It is healing and motivating to know that I am making a positive difference in the lives of people experiencing the negative effects of trauma.

As I said, it is an ongoing process. There are no miraculous cures for PTSD and we both still get triggered sometimes, but we feel that if we stay aware as a family, continue to do the work, reach out to help others, and ask for help when we need it, we will be okay.

If you or a loved one is living with the effects of trauma, PTSD, or OSI, we want you to know that you are not alone and that there is a way forward.

It is a little easier now than back in 2006 when Mike was first diagnosed. So much more is known about PTSD. There is also more awareness throughout the Canadian Forces, although it's still not great. At least now, they know what you're talking about when you mention PTSD. Even outside the military, the stigma persists, but on the whole, there is a greater understanding of PTSD among health professionals and the general public.

Knowledge is power. The more we share our stories and support each other, the more likely we are to overcome the stigma and create more positive outcomes for everyone.

Personal Insights: From Shadows to Light

- You are not alone. In addition to supportive friends and family, there are resources available in your community and online that will help you find the support you need.

- Your recovery from PTSD and other mental health challenges depends on admitting that you have a problem and need help.

- Once you admit that you have a problem, the next step in the process is to ask for help. It is not an easy step and it takes courage, but it is an important part of the process.

- PTSD and mental health issues are not only about you. It is important to recognize that trauma affects everyone in your immediate circle, everyone at work, everyone in your family, all of your loved ones.

- Learning to communicate openly and honestly is essential for recovery. It can take time to acquire the skills you need, but once you do, you will find that your relationships will improve, and your recovery will come quicker. It is helpful if everyone concerned can focus on improving their communication skills.

Kimmy Krochak

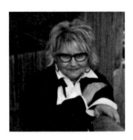 **Kimmy Krochak** gifts the world with her energy, unique charm, humor, and 'sass,' with a slight sprinkle or more of princess (either self-sprinkled or sprinkled from the universe), along with genuine heartfelt kindness and compassion for those she knows and meets. So, it is fitting that when she opened her multi-faceted business as an Energetic Empowerment Consultant & Coach, she called it, none other than "KimmyEnergy."

Kimmy works assisting souls around the world from her current home base in Western Canada. Ego and judgment of other souls has no place, either in her personal life or in her business practice with clients. Down to earth is how she truly is as she speaks her truth to her clients, classes and at events.

Kimmy champions survival, determination and perseverance in the battles against heartache, horrific childhood traumas (physical, mental, emotional, spiritual, and sexual), as well as PTSD. Her gifts allow her to support and assist other souls in making the conscious decision about their own awareness; encouraging individuals to choose to become more than they ever thought possible.

https://www.facebook.com/KimmyEnergy-Potency-of-Choice-752004164848779/

@KimmyEnergyPotencyofChoice

#him2: Supporting Boys to Men

By Kimmy Krochak

Take a moment to imagine the sweetest, most innocent and vulnerable child. This child is about five years old and has just fallen and scraped his knee. Hot, fat tears start pouring down his cheeks and he runs to find his parent for comfort. He is hoping for a hug or even just a look of caring, and a small acknowledgement that everything will be alright.

Instead, his parent barely looks at the scrape before giving the child a hard squeeze on his arm and practically shouts right into his upturned face, "What's the matter with you? It's only a little scrape. You need to learn that *boys don't cry*. Now wipe your face and stop blubbering."

The round-cheeked boy is stunned into silence. All he can do is stand there and numbly rub his cheeks dry and stifle his hiccupping sobs. This little boy has just been initiated into the *boys don't cry* culture that has shut generations of men off from all their emotions. Well, all but one of their emotions. I bet you can guess which emotion men are allowed, and even encouraged, to feel and express whenever they have the need - anger.

Anger is the only emotion that the *boys don't cry* culture allows men to feel. Every other vulnerable emotion – fear, sadness, joy, love – is virtually off-limits to boys and men. If they feel vulnerable at all, they are taught to push it down, stifle it like that little boy's sobs.

Don't be a sissy – be a man. You're not a real man unless you're tough, hard as nails, impervious to weakness. Does that sound familiar?

In my business as multifaceted energetic healer and empowerment coach, I am passionate and dedicated to reversing the damage done to men and women, boys and girls through this culture of emotional oppression. That is at the heart of the #him2 movement.

Let me tell you a story of the moment I was shocked into realizing how powerfully important it is to do this work.

When my son was thirteen years old, he got angry with me because I had brought a friend of his and her family to tears. This family had hired me as a spiritual medium to connect them to their husband/father who had passed away. My job was to use my gifts and abilities as a psychic medium to connect to their loved one's energy on their annual birthday talk to him.

I told my son after the session that his friend and family had been very pleased and happy with the experience. He came to me the next day after school, angry, confused, and frustrated, saying, "Mom, you lied to me! My friend and her family cried and cried after your session. *You said they were happy!*"

I got down so I could be eye to eye with him to explain, "Son, of course they all cried. They all miss and love their father/husband very much. Everything their loved one's spirit told me, I passed on to them. That is a very emotionally intense experience. They had happy *and* sad tears."

My son just stood there in shock listening to me. Something about what I was saying just didn't make sense to him. Then it hit me like one of the harsh cheek-slaps I received in my own childhood: my son didn't understand that crying could *ever* be a *good* thing.

I was immediately reminded of how emotionally unavailable my parents were while I was growing up. I didn't want that for my son, and I would do anything to help him. I asked him, "Son, has someone ever told you that because you are a boy, you shouldn't cry?"

I took a deep breath in anticipation of his answer. I knew I had never oppressed his vulnerable emotions, but perhaps someone else had. "Yes Mom," was all he gave as an answer. For a brief moment, all I could do was bite my lip and keep looking at him until I could find the right words to convey everything that I hoped he could comprehend.

"Oh, my son, it was unkind of someone to have ever said that to you. I am so sorry that happened to you." We talked about how crying is a healthy and necessary release for happy, sad, good, or bad feelings. How important it is that we let those emotions out and not keep them inside our bodies. "Tears are a release of everything that we feel that is not meant to stay inside our hearts, so we shouldn't hold them back, my son."

"Think of it this way: if you don't let your body get rid of your pee and poop you would get a backache and eventually it would cause problems inside of you. You would get so sick that you would need to be hospitalized."

He nodded in agreement and I took a breath. I felt like I had had a near-miss with a future tragedy. Through open, patient dialogue, I undid the damage that someone else had begun. It was a powerful moment that I will never forget.

Through empowerment workshops, I have supported men, women, teens, and children to begin undoing the damage of the *boys don't cry* culture. Through group work and talk therapy they learn that tears are so much more than a bit of shameful wetness on our cheeks.

The physiology of a tear is made up of enzymes, lipids, metabolites and electrolytes. Emotional tears are much different than, say, a tear produced by cutting an onion. Tears from emotional release contain more protein than other tears, which makes them more visible, leaving streaks on the face, while other tears are not as socially noticeable. Emotional tears, you see, are meant to be released and seen by others. They are, by their very chemical nature, made to expose our vulnerability so we can be part of each other's healing.

You may be asking yourself, *how can simply crying make a positive difference to a boy, or even a grown man?* Inside that one tear, each person has access to their own personal data bank, which is able to reference the physical, emotional, mental, spiritual history, and innate awareness. Pushing down these feelings and swallowing our tears adds to our emotional suppression, even at very early ages.

By telling a boy or man at any stage of development that they should not cry, they are robbed of a crucial emotional development process. This is a process whereby we learn to create awareness of our emotions, which leads to positive integration of our emotions into our choices and actions. By learning to connect deeply to self, people are able to honor what is correct for their being, rather than acting from a place of outside opinion or peer pressure. This is a choice as unique to our own being as our own fingerprint.

Less than a month after my son and I had our breakthrough, my husband and I announced to the kids that we were separating. As soon as those words were spoken, my son took my hand and his tears started to fall.

Later, at a family counselling appointment, we shared with our children that mom and dad would have different homes and would be getting a divorce. We all sat together crying and wondering what this new life would be like. My son took my hand, looked me in the eye and said, "Mom, we are all going to be okay."

I still get teared up from thinking of how amazingly mature and emotionally intelligent he was in that moment. In a matter of weeks, he had cracked through the *boys don't cry* culture and was well on his way to emotional freedom.

I am passionate about the #him2 movement not just because my son was told not to cry. It is also because the generational abuse that I endured growing up was partially caused, I believe, by the *boys don't cry* culture. From my very first memories right up to just a few years ago, I have been the recipient of backlash from men who did not have permission to feel and work through those feelings. The backlash took the forms of spiritual, mental, physical, emotional, and sexual abuse.

I believe, right down to my core, that emotional oppression causes abuse, and that empowering men's emotional health will benefit women and men alike.

We all have what I like to call a *motherboard*; a stockpile of every thought and feeling we've had in our lives. Each of us reference this motherboard countless times in a day, subconsciously and consciously; for example, a memory of having someone grab your cheeks as a child and exclaiming how chubby they are. This may cause you to carry roots of that comment inside you. Your motherboard may hold the illusion that you will always be chubby, that when you look in the mirror twenty odd years later you cannot see the cheekbones, you can only see chubby cheeks. The motherboard holds positive and negative experiences equally.

In this way, you can begin to understand how an abuser can be created from the *boys don't cry* culture. Think of that round-cheeked little boy with an upbringing full of emotional suppression, and the encouragement of anger and aggression. He would suffer from emotional neglect and a lack of daily affirmations that build a child's confidence. This sweet child could become withdrawn, which can lead to low self-worth, self-confidence and, most of all, a lack of self-love.

Social institutions and norms don't teach us enough about how to love ourselves, how to appreciate ourselves, and that each and every one of us matters. Instead, we have heard: "Boys don't cry; BIG boys don't cry," and of course, "REAL MEN don't cry!" Who, reading this, has never heard this directed at you or someone you know? Perhaps this has come out of your own mouth without even realizing what you have said.

Another example, often used with girls and women, happens when, in an effort to comfort someone, we say something like, "Sshhh, you don't need to cry over this." You have just told them that their expression of emotion is not valid or warranted for processing their experience. Their emotional release has been shut down, because of your own judgement of how much emotional expression is *too much*. That person may have just lost connection to a small new awareness about their life, or they may have lost the big ah-ha moment that changes their entire existence. Emotional freedom is a personal journey that must be supported and guided instead of being suppressed and judged.

Those boys and men who adhere to the *boys don't cry* culture are automatically cut off from their own natural ability to feel their way through an event or emotion and process it. They often grow up to become men who cannot process their emotions. They are numb or almost numb. They have a motherboard they cannot access.

When the natural response and processing system is stopped, even something as simple as expressing a question or exploring an emotion is stopped as well. We can probably all think of moments when the men in our lives go to extremes of either lashing out or going deep inside themselves to withdrawal. The victims of the *boys don't cry* culture are being conditioned and taught to suppress every emotional event that happens in their lives. They are taught that the simple act of feeling is shameful and worthy of judgment. How completely awful and sad is that?

Suppressing strong emotions is the same thing as ignoring the check engine light when it comes on in your vehicle. If you do not deal with the warning light, the shit will eventually hit the fan. The vehicle will start to make noise, then one day, BAM! Something blows but still, the vehicle somehow drives. It may have a little shimmy or shake, or even a leak, but you still, slowly get to where you are going. You may need gas and oil more often, until eventually the engine seizes up completely.

Our emotions are our engine. Your emotions are just as important to how your body works and processes everything and anything you interact and face all day long. When the emotional engine within us is clogged with suppressed feelings and tears, it will not function properly. It will leak, backfire and eventually stop functioning in a healthy way.

Pause for a moment here to imagine the endless ripples of damage emotional suppression and oppression cause in our lives and our communities. It's a real shit storm, I can tell you! Broken down people everywhere, hurting themselves and each other. We are talking about rage, addictions, violence, lack of respect, poor communication skills, numbness to the people and things that produce pride and joy.

What about the little boys that become soldiers, firemen, police officers, and other first responders? They have traumatic experiences that often haunt their dreams and their day-to-day lives. Imagine them suppressing all of those emotions, not seeking support to process them, just because men are supposed to be tough and not cry. As we have seen in the rates of PTSD, depression and suicide in these professions, emotions must be released in a healthy manner or they will unwittingly be released in unhealthy ways.

This is generational abuse that must end now. We need to find a path to moving beyond emotionally oppressive cultural norms. Most of the people who sustain and pass on the *boys don't cry* culture are parents doing and saying the best they know how in raising their children. If the boys and men in their lives were to fit in and succeed, they needed to conform to the cultural norms of being tough, manly and never crying, period.

Because of the immensity of the problem, I have devoted my professional career to creating and facilitating men's groups for both parolees and those of the general public. In our work together, the men and I are allowed to show our emotions and cry, ask questions or call out for support or help. I support them in being able to step forward in being brave to ask for support in whatever way they need to overcome this, allowing them to reprogram what has happened in the past. This gives them the permission and awareness to come forward without judgment, to create their own change and develop the power to change from being emotional oppressed to emotionally empowered.

With your help we can bring awareness to the #him2 movement and make progress towards ending the *boys don't cry* culture. Through social media, public speaking and community awareness campaigns, together we can undo the damage of men's emotional suppression. Pay attention to the boys and men in your life; how emotionally free are they? Do they paint their lives with the full palette of emotional colors? Or are they only painting with red and black? Boycott media that perpetuates the *boys don't cry* culture and support those media sources that demonstrate men's emotional freedom. Don't stand by silently while a boy is told not to cry; speak up and support him. The #metoo movement has done so much for girls and women, let's speak out for #him2. It will benefit all of society in the end.

In case you are still not convinced that the #him2 movement is worth your support, here's a vivid real-life example. No one in Canada or around the world will ever forget where they were when the Humboldt Broncos bus crashed in 2018. Think of all those people, on the bus, and off. The families, friends, team support staff, classmates, first responders, medical staff, drivers and so on. The circles of impact extend far and wide. Can you feel even a glimpse of that? So many lives affected, so many tears that needed to be released, so many emotions that needed support.

What would happen if we, as a society, commanded that all those who were involved in or affected by the crash must not cry or show emotion? What if all those affected suppressed every tear, every bit of grief, and sadness. What kind of a mess would we have on our hands? Can you feel how powerfully negative that would be for our society? And conversely, how deeply positive and enriching taking a #him2 stance would be for everyone? This is an example how suppressing emotions, regardless of your gender, is so damaging to one's being.

I'll never forget the day I began to understand the positive impact my work with men's emotional freedom was starting to have in my community. While shopping one day, a shopper in the store called me over to share some good news. One of her employees had recently taken my emotional empowerment workshop. She shared with me how dramatically different her employee's attitude and interpersonal skills were at work since then. Where there used to be hot-tempered, aggressive, over-talking behaviours, the employee was now contributing meaningfully at staff meetings and not having outbursts of negativity. There is no better compliment than hearing from a business owner about the positive changes they see in their workplaces after my workshops.

The employee in question (for privacy's sake let's call him Luke), told me later how much easier it is for him to step back from his anger after working with me. Luke said before there was no thinking, only reacting. Now he understands himself. He knows how to tune in and then choose to live from a more level-headed, peaceful mindset. Making room for the vulnerable emotions in his life has eased the pressure on the anger and aggression as the only mode of expression. One workshop attendee at a time, boys and men are untying themselves from the bindings of emotional suppression.

We are gifting them not only permission to feel but also to make the choice to create change for more abundance in their lives. They can finally begin to heal what is deep down, dark, and painful for them. Through this process, men begin to live, feel, and believe that they are worthy, confident and proud to be emotional beings. They live this truth in their own mind, heart, soul, and right through their own skin. They will be walking around saying, "Bow chicka-wow-wow, look at me! Aren't I great?!"

Through emotional empowerment, men stop feeling like robots that just work, take out the garbage, drive the kids to practice, and express one or two emotional states. Men begin to understand themselves. They begin to feel things more deeply, and believe that it's good to express their feelings *and their vulnerabilities*.

I ask you to pledge with me through the #him2 movement to support baby boys, teens, and men in their journeys to emotional freedom. Next time you're with a male in your life of any age or role, pay attention to their level of emotional freedom. If you notice them starting to withdraw or have a behavior change, try placing a gentle hand on their shoulder to create a safe place for them. Then try something like this –

"May I ask a question? I have noticed (and/or feel) that something is off. Is there some way I can support you?"

It is very possible that the boy or man you are talking to may look at you like you're an alien, but that's okay. Just stay still and let them see that you really mean it. They may not open up right then, but they will begin to see that you are a person who wants them to be emotionally free - and that is just the start of the #him2 movement's impact.

My wish for all the boys and men, and the girls and women in their lives, is that everyone knows their feelings are valid and allowed. I wish for every age and gender to have self-love and the ability to ask for, and accept, emotional support when they need it. With your help, we can create a generation of boys and men who will never be told that *boys don't cry.*

Personal Insights: From Shadows to Light

- You are enough.

- You are worthy to be emotionally and mentally free to break old patterns and habits.

- Asking for support does not make you weak.

- Your possibilities for abundance and peace are there for you.

- Keep going in your search for support. You will know and feel the "click" when you find the right source of support.

Cinnamon Cranston

Cinnamon Cranston is a University of Regina and Mount Royal College graduate, a Reiki practitioner, and a Registered Massage Therapist who specializes in the Rosen Method.

Informed by her personal experience and her own quest for peace and healing, Cinnamon's 20-year journey through the health and wellness field has focused on treating and overcoming the effects of trauma. After exploring a number of modalities, she discovered the importance of the body in the recovery process. In 2008, she knew she was home when her search led her to the Rosen Method, which seeks to access the unconscious in the body and to integrate it.

Today, Cinnamon is a certified a Rosen Method Bodywork Practitioner with a private practice in Edmonton, Alberta, called The Mindful Body. She is also a Rosen Method Workshop Teacher and Rosen Method Movement Teacher.

www.themindfulbody.ca
@mindfulbody_yeg
@cinnamoncranston

Lionheart

By Cinnamon Cranston

I have always been the kind of person who never gave up on the possibility that there is more to life than suffering, even though life gave me every reason to believe exactly the opposite. I experienced more than my share of suffering early in life. Before the age of eight, I had experienced the abandonment of my mother during my parents' acrimonious separation, sexual interference from a babysitter, a near-fatal car accident, and the severe neglect that comes with having an alcoholic single parent mother. When I was nine years old, my mother quit drinking and remarried. My quality of life improved significantly, but I would still have to endure sexual and physical abuse from a family member and a boyfriend. In the absence of any kind of emotional support, I learned to live in a state of collapse for my own self-preservation. Hidden deep within me, though, my spirit had most definitely not lost the will to fight. From there, it pushed me forward, despite the intense fear I lived with daily. I never gave up the search and the longing for a different way to live.

***

Despite becoming a well-educated twenty-something and an entrepreneur with my own business, I had also become an alcoholic. I was racked with fear and depression on the inside, despite having a brave and competent face on the outside. Some of the most important first steps I took toward healing, included admitting that I was suffering from alcoholism at the age of twenty-eight, and taking the necessary action to begin my recovery from addiction. I come from a long line of Irish Catholic alcoholics; the disease had destroyed families on my mother's side for many generations. I also knew that I was suffering from a wide range of other dysfunctional behaviors as a result of my early-life experiences. I sought help and began my healing in the rooms of twelve-step recovery. As my life started to change for the better, I got married to my partner and we started a family. With a year and a half of recovery under my belt, I thought my past was long behind me, until, one day, it became undeniable that my childhood experiences were still affecting my capacity to respond appropriately in the present moment.

At the time, I had recently moved to Edmonton. I was a stay-at-home mother, pregnant with my second child and caring for my eighteen-month-old son. My mother, who lived in Regina, Saskatchewan, had been going through chemotherapy treatment for what turned out to be terminal ovarian cancer. The stress of losing my mother, being pregnant, and parenting a toddler in a city where I didn't know anyone, was overwhelming. To add to the stress, my husband traveled a lot for work, leaving me home alone with my son for up to a week at a time. All of this acted like a pressure cooker inside me. While I looked very together and highly functional on the outside, inside I was a mess of fear and anxiety; lost in the panic of trying to get it right, trying to be perfect.

Then one evening I had a breakdown. My husband was away on a business trip and my son and I were alone at home. My son was standing on the change table, screaming at the top of his lungs. I had just changed his diaper and he was tired and anxious.

Unfortunately, I did not respond well to his protests. Something in me snapped and I lost control of my emotions. I began to yell at him to stop crying. I was hysterically angry. My son in turn became more and more hysterical. I kept yelling. He kept screaming and crying. It was an awful scene. Then I had a moment of what I can only call grace. I was able to pause and hear myself, hear how crazy I sounded. I looked at my son and saw how scared he was of me. My heart sank and my eyes welled up with tears. I felt like I was the most terrible person in the world.

I knew in that moment that I had fallen far from the person I wanted to be. I immediately picked him up and comforted him. I told him how sorry I was for yelling at him. Right then, I knew without a doubt that there was something going on inside me that I could not fix on my own, or with the self-help, twelve-step approach I had taken thus far. I knew I needed professional help, and my guilt over my behavior motivated me to begin psychotherapy.

***

At first, psychotherapy was very helpful. It helped me understand how unsafe my past experiences had been and how they had shaped me. However, when we began to get into the *feelings* connected with my past, psychotherapy began to fall short. I would often leave my session in a dissociated state, remaining too long in the feelings of the past. The imaginary safe spaces and hypnosis we used during therapy were not enough to alleviate the intense fear and anxiety I was experiencing between sessions; I struggled to function in my daily life as a stay-at-home mother. As a trained massage therapist and Reiki practitioner, I knew that my body was also suffering, and I asked my therapist if there was anything I could do about it. She recommended that I see a counsellor who practiced Integrative Body Psychotherapy (IBP), a type of psychotherapy that treats the somatic (physical), psychological, and spiritual nature of a human being. I preferred this approach to psychotherapy because I felt much more supported as a 'whole' person.

IBP focuses on body awareness and breath during the sharing of experiences and emotions. This approach helped me immensely. I no longer left my therapy sessions in a dissociated state because the therapy also worked with the sensation of boundary, as well as spiritual replenishment. I came to understand that I had Post Traumatic Stress Disorder (PTSD) from my numerous early childhood traumas, which had been activated by becoming a mother myself. I began to heal a lot of my dysfunctional behaviors. I learned to re-parent myself and be in my body with my feelings by using a physical sense of boundary along with imaginal resources to ground me when the feelings got too overwhelming. I have a deep respect for IBP methodology, as it laid a solid foundation for me to grow and dramatically improved my capacity to have healthy relationships.

After seven years of IBP treatment, I began to experience symptoms of anxiety and panic again. I could not resolve them with the tools my counsellor had given me, and it was affecting my quality of life. There were still times when I would need to retreat from my life and lie on the couch for several days to recover from an episode of panic or rage. Even though I was able to manage my intense emotional reactions (not projecting them outward onto other people), I was still caught in re-experiencing those emotions with no apparent connection to their cause. I found this very disheartening. After all of the great healing work I had done in therapy, it only took a moment to trigger my past feelings and bring great distress into my body. I was angry and frustrated at my lack of control over these episodes, and I was determined to find a way out of the trauma cycle.

My therapist advised me to try Rosen Method Bodywork (RMB), a form of somatic therapy that uses gentle, present touch, and words to access unconscious emotional memory within the body. She explained that the particular type of touch that RMB offered would help me to access unconscious memory within the body in a way that IBP could not, and that this kind of therapy would help me heal from the trauma I had experienced. The idea that there was even more trauma buried in my past frightened me. I wasn't sure I wanted to remember more. Although I had worked with the body for years as a massage therapist, letting someone touch me in a way that would help me connect to my unconscious feelings and experiences, worried me. Would I be safe with this person? How could they support me if they weren't a counsellor or a psychotherapist? Trust has never been easy for me, and it took another year for me to open up to trying an RMB session. Eventually, my desire to heal won over my fear of trying something new.

***

During my first Rosen Method Bodywork session, I was amazed at its directness and effectiveness in helping me to connect with my body. I began to feel new sensations that I had never noticed before. Without knowing anything about my story, the practitioner was remarkably insightful and knew things about me, such as how strong and tough I had been growing up. This was a relief, but it was shocking at the same time. Finally, somebody understood, somebody really could see how hard I was working to be here, to be safe. She could also see my collapse, the part of me that didn't want to be here. As she spoke and touched me with supportive and listening hands, I began to feel just how hard my body was working to protect me.

At one point in the session, I felt an intense sadness as she worked on my chest. I let the feelings emerge. A memory came to me of a near-death experience I'd had when I was five years old. I had almost died in a severe roll-over in the Drumheller valley. I remembered and felt the experience of being in the space between life and death. I was looking down at the truck wreck where it had fallen in the valley below, desperately not wanting to go back there, but knowing I had to. I had never experienced this memory before. I wasn't alone in that in-between place. There were other beings or souls around me, and they were telling me that it wasn't my time yet. I knew I had to return to the world, but I decided that I wouldn't go back all the way. At this point in the session, I could feel the frozen stillness of my death pose in my body. I became aware of the part of me that had always been living just outside of me, more in the unseen world than in this one. I had lived with one foot out the door my whole life, ready to die because being here was just too painful.

Even after all the years of therapy, my body was still holding on to so much and, until that moment, I had had no idea. The practitioner gently invited me to come back into my being, to explore what it felt like to be in the present. Her gentle, supportive touch was reassuring and helped me to reconnect to my body in way I had never before experienced. I felt myself breathe with a full breath for the first time that I could remember. I felt like I had truly landed in my body at long last. The session was a breakthrough moment for me: it was the first time I had come out of my collapse. My body could discern on some level that it was safe to be here and that I could now choose to be here. At that moment, I knew that this was the work I had long been waiting for. I signed up for training. Three and a half years later I became a certified practitioner of Rosen Method Bodywork.

During training, we students were invited to listen deeply within ourselves and to connect with each other, essence to essence, touching from the heart without any expectations, and using words that came from within our own experiences, not our analytical minds. I deeply appreciated this type of connection. It was what I had longed for my whole life. The personal growth I experienced during my RMB training was immeasurable. As a student, I was required to receive a specific number of sessions myself. During each one of these, a different emotional memory arose and always surprised me. Some of the most difficult feelings that came up were shame-based feelings of being bad, terrible, and unlovable. I learned that when terrible things happen to us, we often come to believe that we are terrible ourselves. With the practitioner's supportive, compassionate touch, I could allow these feelings to be felt and spoken, knowing it was safe enough now to do so. In this way, my body learned to integrate past experiences, rather than reliving or repressing them. My body relaxed, more deeply than ever before, and I felt more present inside my body. I came to trust the support of the connection I had with the practitioner. My chronic panic and anxiety left me completely. I gradually felt whole from the inside out. I developed a new way of being within myself and within the moment. I could be *with* uncomfortable feelings, and not be *overwhelmed* by them. I was no longer trapped in the cycle of trauma.

***

Rosen Method Bodywork was the missing link to my recovery and I passionately wanted to share it with the world. I thought everyone should be aware of this method and was frustrated that no one knew about it. I became an advocate for RMB, writing articles for *Mosaic Magazine*, posting to my own blog, and talking about the work I do with anyone who would listen. I felt passionately that this therapy was so effective in helping people heal from their trauma that it deserved to be better known to professionals and covered by medical insurance. I believe that people should have a choice in what they want for mental health care and they shouldn't have to be wealthy get the care that they need.

In the last year of my training, the neuroscience behind why RMB (and other somatic modalities) worked, exploded onto the scene. Science had begun to understand what happens to the body when it has experienced trauma, as well as what the brain and body needed to fully recover from it. Alan Fogel, a Ph.D. in Psychology and an RMB teacher, came to teach at my school. He had just published his book, *The Psychophysiology of Self-Awareness: Rediscovering the Lost Art of Body Sense* and talked about the science behind somatic therapies. I felt relieved to have scientific evidence to support what we had been taught. I later used this new information when advocating RMB to professionals who relied on scientific, evidence-based research to validate new therapies. Frustrated at how uninformed most health care workers were (and still are) about trauma, I focused most of my efforts on informing people about what it is and how complete healing and resolution requires a somatic approach that accesses the deeper sensory parts of the brain. Trauma cannot be healed by using only a cognitive or talk therapy approach.

My healing journey has been ongoing. While establishing my private practice in Edmonton as an RMB Practitioner, I continued to support my own healing through both Rosen Method Bodywork and Somatic Experiencing®, a therapy similar to RMB, founded by renowned trauma therapist Peter Levine. I believe it is important for me to carry on with my own healing process, ever learning. Even now, I continue to recover emotional memories and integrate experiences of early childhood trauma. One of those experiences was of a time when my parents separated; I was three years old. The memory came through gradually, over the course of several treatments. It first manifested as a deep sense of being frozen and unsafe throughout my entire body. I felt in my body, a general sense of being in extreme life-threatening danger, which progressed to an awareness of being in an intense, hysterical rage. I then had the sensation of being choked, being very still and shut down, and then being unconscious. I sensed that my father was there with me and that he was in a rage. I remembered the terror of not being able to breathe, of his rage, of my fear, and the sudden feeling of being rendered unconscious.

My interpretation of these somatic memories is an interesting part of my healing and learning process. While I had recovered some very potent sensory memories, there were still many unknown facts about this time in my life. What I had to go on, was a story my mother had told me of how my father, in a rage, had taken me from her for two weeks after catching her cheating on him at a party. In addition to this narrative, I have also always had a visceral, physical response of fear and anxiety around my father that I could never explain; it has made it difficult for me to trust him. As a result, I interpreted my somatic memories with the explanation that my father must have been angry with me for being hysterical over missing my mother and that he must have been the cause of my choking sensation. I held on to this interpretation for several years and chose to avoid a relationship with him.

Recently, I had the opportunity to ask my father about this time in our lives and I heard the love and kindness in his voice. Finally, after years of somatic therapy, I felt healed enough within my body so that I no longer experienced terror and anxiety when speaking with him. I shared with him all of my sensory memories and how I had interpreted them. Then I asked him to share what he remembered. My father said that I was indeed hysterical, inconsolable at my mother's leaving. He then explained that he had gone home, after catching my drunk mother being unfaithful. When my mother arrived home the next morning, they had a row and he asked her to leave, giving her two weeks to find a new place and get herself together. He remembered trying to comfort me after my mother left, but it didn't work. He said that at no time did he ever use force to stop me from crying. He did, however, remember that I was crying so hard that I could not catch my breath and that I was choking. Eventually, I cried myself to sleep. He said that I was a very astute child and that I would have either heard the argument or felt the anger that he was working hard to contain. Later, he took me to my grandmother's where I was upset again, crying that my mother had run away.

Hearing my father's account of events had a remarkable effect on me. All of my sensory memories fit with his version of the facts. I had independently come up with a different interpretation to explain my feelings, but his story seemed believable. My instincts told me that I could trust his account, that he was telling the truth as far as he could remember it. My father had been angry but not with me. He had been trying to protect me. I choked from my own tears, not from being choked. I was terrified and angry and helpless. Eventually my body shut down all the big feelings and I passed out asleep. I had associated my father with the terrifying feelings of abandonment because he was the one I was left with. We had shared the experience of abandonment together, albeit differently. It also made sense to me that my mother had come up with a tale to assuage her own guilt and suffering for causing a separation between us. This experience has taught me that the narrative or story of my past can change, and that it is important to recognize that the mind likes to fill in the gaps between sensory memories, sometimes incorrectly. I have learned that it is important to keep going, renegotiating the past within the present experience under the care of an experienced practitioner.

Today, I find myself free to be creative in ways I would never have let myself be in the past. I have reached a level of trust and intimacy in my relationships that I had always dreamed of but never knew how to achieve. Most importantly, I have developed a deep and abiding trust in my soul as I experience it within my body. It is this trust that allows me to do the work I do with others, helping them to experience the same freedom.

***

Looking back on my path to recovery, it is clear to me that the best combination for healing from trauma is both a top-down trauma-informed approach (psychotherapy, talk therapy, cognitive behavioral therapy) and a bottom-up trauma-informed approach (RMB, Somatic Experiencing®). If I had been able to receive help from a trauma-informed counselor and a somatic bodywork therapist from the beginning, my recovery might not have taken so long. But this option was not available to me then as it would be now. Fortunately, although there are still too few well-trained, trauma-informed, somatic bodywork therapists, there are now several trauma-informed talk therapists where I live in Edmonton (some of whom also work with touch). While the quality of care is improving within the therapeutic field, there are still major issues with health coverage, continuing education on trauma for front-line health and mental health professionals, and the education of future somatic trauma therapists. Right now, the education path for therapies such as RMB is a long and costly process, with few options for training that often require travel. It would be nice to see it become more mainstream, offered at universities or colleges as part of a somatic psychology discipline, and recognized by health care providers nationally.

There is also a need for reform in the mental health system, so that everyone can have access to a more comprehensive range of healing options. An ideal system would include a fully funded, culturally sensitive, team-assessment approach for anyone wanting or requiring mental health treatment. The team would include trauma-informed care providers trained in a variety of approaches, not just conventional medical doctors and psychiatrists. Patients would be consulted and have choices around the type of care they receive.

Collectively, these reforms to the mental health and tertiary education systems would contribute to a more caring society in which everyone would be fortunate enough to have access to the same treatment as I did, as well as any other modalities that would best suit their needs, regardless of their socio-economic status. This is my dream. The work I do is now a practice of loving gratitude for having had the opportunity to heal from my trauma, and for being able to use this knowledge and experience to assist others with their healing.

Personal Insights: From Shadows to Light

- I now know that the physical and emotional suffering I have experienced as an adult is deeply connected to what happened to me in childhood and that it *is* possible for me to heal from those experiences.

- I have learned that pain was something I experienced, it is not who I was or who I am.

- While healing early childhood developmental trauma it was important for me to develop and invite nurturing and protective resources for my inner child.

- Embodied self-awareness is what connects me to my core essence; not analytical thinking.

- I have learned to replace judgment with curiosity. Cultivating a practice of mindfulness and a non-judgmental view of my inner experiences has been important for maintaining my mental health and well-being.

- Sometimes I have had to play dead to live. This doesn't mean that my spirit ever gave up, it means that I was actually being the bravest I could ever be. This shift in perspective released me from shame.

- I do have the capacity to shift out of survival mode and cultivate well-being within my body.

- Trauma is a part of life. Everyone will, at some point in their life, experience trauma. What makes a person resilient in the face of traumatic experience is their capacity for embodied self-awareness and self-regulation.

- The healing journey is like a spiral; often we find ourselves at a familiar part of our story, yet we are healing a different aspect of it. A deeper level of healing happens with each pass around the circle, ever spiraling us forward towards our true essence.

Cindy Klamn-Conway

In her life, **Cindy** has faced many challenges, but never allowed fear to knock her down. She thrives on her strength and positivity to turn all situations into life lessons. Cindy is a natural born medium who chooses to use her gift to bring happiness and peace into the lives 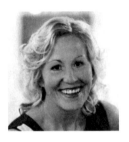 of others who may need support or answers in the darkest times of their lives. Cindy brings a unique blend of passion, honesty and equality, and shares it with her community and family. She has the ability to embrace people as they genuinely are, without judgment or flaws, which allows for her true authentic self to shine through.

When she was 35 years old, Cindy and her husband packed up and moved to Calgary where they raised their three beautiful children. Cindy enjoys her time with her dogs and spends most of her free time connecting with family and friends. She also spends her time volunteering with the grassroots organization, I Belong Bags, where she helps children-in-crisis transition into new homes and provides them with basic necessities and comfort items.

Cindy now offers wellness treatments at her studio in Calgary, and also offers the healing clarity of Medium services to her clients.

https://www.facebook.com/AbovetheCloudsWithCindy/

I Choose to Rise Above

By Cindy Klamn-Conway

Growing up with alcoholic parents made for an extremely abusive and neglectful home. Most of the memories I have from childhood are of witnessing my parents fighting constantly, of living in unclean conditions with mice and dirt everywhere, and of neighbors and friends gathering in our home late at night because it was always open for people to come in and drink. Eventually the alcohol and the partying became more important than us, so we were often left to fend for ourselves. My mother left when I was five years old. She would still show up periodically, more to upset the apple cart than anything else. My dad was physically there, but because of the alcohol, he wasn't really available to parent us. I did have other sources of support that my siblings didn't have; I had my spirit companions. I later realized that they were my protectors, but as a child I didn't think of them that way and I didn't foresee the important role they would play in my life. They were just my friends. I talked to them; spent time with them. I had no idea that I was *channelling* them, much less what a rare gift I had. They were just part of my normal life.

Feelings and communication were not my dad's forte. He had his own approach to life and problem-solving. He taught me a lot of practical "guy" skills, like putting up drywall or changing the oil in my car, but not about what it meant to be a woman in this world. I learned nothing about sexuality, setting healthy boundaries, or what to expect from boys; it just didn't come up. There were a lot of "uncles" who would come over to the house to drink. Some would touch me inappropriately or make me sit on their laps. I knew I didn't like it, but I had no context for understanding my feelings of discomfort. No one ever said anything or put a stop to it, so I just thought it was normal. Consequently, at the age of seventeen, I was not only completely naïve and unprepared for the adult world; my sense of boundaries was fluid at best. I also had no personal experience with alcohol, having made a conscious decision not to drink.

The summer before I turned eighteen, I went out with a girlfriend. She suggested we go to a lounge, which seemed like a fun adventure. Up to that point I hadn't really had a social life; I was too busy trying to keep my dad sober. It was a losing battle, but when I was old enough, I stayed close to home and looked for ways to keep him from drinking.

Getting into the bar was surprisingly easy; we were never asked for identification. The bar was dark, we walked in and sat at a round table in the middle of the room. When the waitress came to take our order, I had no idea what to drink, so I ordered the only cocktail I knew of- a screwdriver. When it came, I didn't like it much, but my dad had always told me that a drink was something you always finished. Whether it was in a bottle or in a glass, once you started, you *had* to finish, so I did. We sat, and talked, and giggled like we hadn't a care in the world. We felt like sophisticated grown-ups.

Not long after we sat down, four men seated at a nearby table started talking to us. I couldn't believe it — *A man, interested in me?* No one had ever shown interest in *me* before. It was new and, frankly, exhilarating. For the first time in my life, I felt pretty. When they complimented me, it made me feel like I was somebody worth talking to. If I had any walls, they came down almost immediately and I lost all my inhibitions and fears.

The men bought us so many drinks I lost count. In all honesty, I don't remember a lot of detail, but I know that when the music came on, we danced. It was so exciting that someone wanted to dance with me. *Me!* When they complimented my dancing, I remember feeling so elegant and beautiful. As the night progressed, one of the men suggested that we go back to their apartment to have a party. I had never been in someone's apartment before, and I had never been invited to an "adult" party, which made the thought of going even more exciting.

The choice I made to drink that day had taken away my ability to make rational decisions. Had I not been drinking, I would never have agreed to leave with men I had just met. I may not yet have had a good sense of boundaries, but I did know that much. But, consuming so many drinks blinded me to the danger; the alcohol was making all of the decisions for me. Under its influence, my girlfriend and I felt that, because we had spent so much time with these men, we knew them pretty well. Whether or not to accept their invitation was an easy decision: it was an absolute "yes." We got into the car with two of the men, but the other two begged us not to go. They went so far as to try pulling us out of the vehicle. But we didn't understand why they were trying to get us out, so we stayed in the car. We didn't understand that they were trying to save us.

When we arrived at the apartment, I felt comfortable and at ease. I was very excited about the attention I was getting. I don't remember the men making any sexual advances before we got to the apartment, but my only experience with men had been with the drunk "uncles" at our house when I was a child. Given that experience, and having never been taught about sex or safety, how was I to know? My "uncles" had made me uncomfortable, but these men weren't like that. They were worse.

By the time I realized what was happening it was too late. I stepped out onto the porch and, in the blink of an eye, the nice man who had followed me out transformed into a monster. He attacked me, grabbed me, dragged me by the hair, beat me, and pulled me inside. I could hear my friend screaming in another room. I was suddenly in Hell. He dragged me into a bedroom and brutally raped me. In a single moment my innocence was gone.

After the man got off me, he stood and said, "Stay there and don't move a fuckin' inch." He went out to the living room across the hall. That's when I heard the "click." It reminded me of when my dad lit a cigarette. In that moment, I knew that those two or three seconds it would take for him to put down the lighter and come back, would be my only chance to escape. I leapt up and ran out of the room, down the hall, to the front door (it wasn't locked), and down the stairs to the street. I was half naked and barefoot. I remember running, and running, and running, so fast and so hard that I couldn't breathe. I had no idea where I was or how to get home.

Then I saw a railyard. We lived near train tracks. I just headed that way hoping to get my bearings. Instead, I found myself in what looked like a homeless camp. I was physically exposed and in a state of panic. Then the catcalls began, and I was grabbed, groped, and almost gang raped by several men. Time stood still. I screamed and kicked and fought so hard to get out of there. Then I felt a presence around me and somehow, I managed to get away. My feet were so sore I could hardly walk but I kept going. I don't remember how I managed to get home, but I woke up in my bed the next morning, disoriented. Part of me wondered if it had really happened at all or if it was a nightmare. To this day, I believe that the presence I had felt was one of my guardian angels stepping in to save me.

The guilt was awful. I never talked to, or even saw, my girlfriend again. I had heard her screaming. It was hard to live with myself, knowing I had left her behind in that apartment; I still don't what had happened to her. The guilt only compounded my shame for having been raped. I did not tell *anyone* what happened to me that night. How could I? *It was all my fault. I had brought it on myself. I only had myself to blame.*

***

Six or seven weeks after the rape, I was not feeling very well. I went to the doctor and told him that I was feeling nauseated. I thought I might have the flu because I wasn't getting any better. Initially he didn't ask me any questions. He didn't even ask me if I was sexually active. When I eventually told him about the rape, he didn't care. He just told me I had to get a pregnancy test done. I remember crying and saying, "Why do I have to do a test when I didn't do anything wrong?" My education on reproductive matters was so limited that I thought a pregnancy test was a written test. It felt like I was being punished, even though I hadn't done anything wrong.

The results came back positive. I was pregnant, but I didn't know how it had happened. I didn't understand what had caused a pregnancy and it made no sense to me. I can't quite explain it, but I literally did not understand what pregnant meant. I was a virgin before the attack, I had never been given "the sex talk," and I had no idea where babies came from. I had seen pregnant women before, but it still didn't click. I was so confused; I just couldn't wrap my head around what was happening.

When I finally understood that I was going to have a baby, I knew I couldn't keep it. The thought of putting it up for adoption did cross my mind, but I was not equipped to make an informed decision. In my muddled thinking, I couldn't imagine the child growing up without its mother, like I had. And, knowing nothing of confidentiality issues, I couldn't bear the thought of the child finding out it was the product of a violent rape. My heart just broke. I made the only decision I felt I could at the time: I chose to end the pregnancy. It wasn't an easy choice, but I couldn't see that I had any other option.

In those days, abortion was barely legal and subject to medical approval. A few days later, I went before a board of four men, I think they were doctors. It was a demeaning, embarrassing, humiliating experience. They knew I had been raped but they made it very clear that they were doing me a favor because I was obviously promiscuous. They treated me as if I had asked to be raped and did it all the time. They accused me of having a drinking problem. They also made it clear they didn't want this decision on their shoulders because it would hurt the hospital's reputation.

Those four men were relentless in their judgment and their cruelty was only too apparent. They called me unspeakable names and told me what a "despicable girl" I was, over and over again, for hours. I didn't understand much of what they were saying, which only added to my confusion. It was a horrendous experience, and I went through it alone, with zero support. I had no choice, there was no one in my life I could rely on.

The board decided it would reluctantly allow the abortion. I was told that it could take place at their hospital but that I could not tell anyone, and had to register in the morning for a D&C, not an abortion. When I left that room, the feelings I had been holding inside came crashing down on me all at once. I wanted to walk in front of a bus. I couldn't ask for help because I was too ashamed and still too scared to tell anyone about what had happened to me. No one would understand. I was all alone.

For years, I relived the rape in my head. My thoughts were filled with questions: *Why did this happen to me? What did I do to deserve this?* And then, of course, there were all the "what ifs" that scared me to the core: *What if it happens again? What if someone finds out what happened? What if…?* To say that it was something I just put in the back of my mind and moved on from, would be a lie. Soon, the emotional trauma started to affect me physically, it began literally to eat me up inside — I developed severe stomach ulcers from the stress and from failing to properly deal with the emotional fallout of my experience.

Despite the pain and trauma, I held fast to the belief that there is a reason for everything; a conviction that helped me persevere whenever I felt like giving up. Without support, I had to become my own cheerleader. I'm not going to tell you that it was easy because it wasn't. The weight of what had happened to me would build up in the background sometimes and I would "lose it" over the smallest thing. I was drowning in my own shame.

I engaged in a lot of extremely negative self-talk and there were times when I behaved irrationally. I was reasonably social at work and I had friends, but then I would isolate myself in the evenings, stay home, locked away. I didn't realize that I wasn't dealing with the trauma of the rape and its aftermath. I was extremely sad and very lonely. I was afraid of every little noise in the dark and of everyone around me. I was nervous all of the time. Deep down, I wanted someone, anyone, to help me, but where could I turn? I couldn't afford professional help and I wasn't going to tell my friends or family. I told myself, *You made a choice to do it alone, so do it alone. Stand tall, shoulders back, and head held high. You can do this!* I would give myself a good kick in the butt, and off I would go ploughing through my day.

I forced myself to put on a façade of easy-going confidence, which came naturally to me because of my childhood. From the outside I looked like I was on top of my game; nobody could tell that on the inside I was dying. Nobody knew that the minute I walked out to my car alone from work or the gym, the fear of being raped again was paralyzing. Every time I approached my car, my heart would race, and my hands would shake. I would look under the car just in case someone was there. I would check the backseat in case someone was there. I would get into my car with the speed of an Olympic athlete and quickly lock the doors once I was inside.

It was only then that my heart would start to slow down and my hands would stop shaking. But then, when I reached my destination, I would have to get out of my car and the "what ifs" would start all over again. I remember that one time, I bought a knife for protection and held it in my hand hiding it from view with the blade facing up against my wrist. I made my way from the car to my house. I was shaking so violently that by the time I got to the door, I had cuts all over my arm where the blade had crossed my skin. Fear had me in its grip and I had no idea how to deal with it.

Even my home wasn't safe anymore. My sister lived next door and I would have her kids meet me at my house to check all of the closets and every room, just to make sure no one was inside. After they were gone, every little noise caused my heart to race. My mind would create the most vivid and horrifying scenarios. I knew I needed help, but I still didn't know how I could ever tell another living soul what had happened to me.

Choosing to keep the truth about the attack and the ensuing emotions hidden instead of dealing with them, allowed the darkness to take over. Like a child pulling the blankets over her head to keep the monsters away, my attempts to hide what I was going through only added to my fears. They grew exponentially.

I never formally dealt with my mental health, but I did find a way through, eventually. It wasn't easy but I have been able to find a measure of peace and a new purpose in life.

My recovery began when I decided to focus on my physical health, first. I knew I needed to rebuild my psyche and learn to live without constant fear, but I just felt unable to face the trauma. I started exercising like crazy to pass the time. I worked out three times a day and played several sports on top of that. The activity kept me busy, so I didn't have time to think. At the same time, though, it started to have a beneficial effect on my overall mindset and mental health. I slowly became stronger on all levels.

I then met and married a partner I could trust, and I surrounded myself with reliable friends who have supported me through my recovery. And, of course, I had my spirits who, even in the darkest times, never abandoned me. These beneficent spirits were not only my friends, they were- and are- my guides. They were instrumental in getting me through my own personal nightmare and gave me a new lease on life. Once I also understood that I could help others as an intuitive spiritual guide/medium by channelling their deceased loved ones, I knew I had found my true purpose in life. Today I have my own meaningful, heart-centred practice, Above the Clouds, helping others overcome their own life challenges.

Although it would not be the last life-altering challenge I would go through, I believe the rape has shaped me into the person I am today. I can stand before you and tell you everything is under control, not because it is always easy, but because I have chosen the path forward rather than staying stuck in the past. I have surrounded myself with a reliable support system, and I have found meaning in my life: my family, my practice, my health. My husband and I are teaching our daughters and our son to be aware of their surroundings, to make smart choices, to set personal boundaries, to understand the importance of body autonomy, and to have respect for others. I feel good about the job we are doing with them.

It has been a long journey to physical and emotional recovery, but like I said, I believe everything happens for a reason. The rape has propelled me forward and fuelled my desire to help others, which in turn has given me the power to tackle my own emotional issues, including the negative self-talk.

By sharing my story, I am making a conscious choice to take the power away from my rapist, take control of my life, and empower others. My hope is that by shining a light on my story and bringing it to women who have been through similar trauma, I can help them realize that they are not alone; that they can not only survive their experience, but learn to thrive and enjoy life again. Together, we work to heal their injured souls, lift the blankets off their heads, and leave the darkness behind.

Personal Insights: From Shadows to Light

- The rape was not my fault: I take full responsibility for my choices that night, but that does not mean the rape is my fault. That man had no right to violate me regardless of the circumstances.

- The doctors who judged me for my rape were wrong and disrespectful. Their behavior was unprofessional and unforgivable. Their treatment of me has forever changed my perception of medical professionals.

- If you are struggling with similar trauma, don't go through it alone. Although I didn't have the luxury of accessing mental health services as we have today, I'm not sure I would have reached out, even if I had. I now realize that I could have saved myself years of pain if I had gotten help. Please reach out to someone; anyone!

- Safety starts with each of us. I wasn't old enough or equipped to make good decisions on that fateful day. I now know better: I don't drink, I set healthy boundaries, and I trust my intuition when a situation feels off. I have also chosen to learn how to physically protect myself, and to encourage young girls to learn self-defence.

- There is a reason for everything. I have been given the opportunity to turn this horrific experience into something positive, and that has become my life's work. I take every opportunity I am given to share my story and what I have learned with young girls.

- It is important for each of us to own our power. By sharing my story, I took my power back; you can do the same.

- We are never truly alone. I didn't have support from anyone in my life during this time, but something inside of me kept reassuring me that I was not alone. I am surrounded not only by friendly spirits but also by angels who protect and guide me. I believe everyone has guardian angels and spirit guides around them. Listen for them; call on them. They are there to guide and protect you.

Vireo Karvonen

Vireo Karvonen is a licensed Belief Re-patterning® Practitioner and Sacred Sexuality Coach who has been supporting and empowering women for well over a decade.

Vireo's deep-rooted desire to positively impact others goes back to 1996, when she completed her Master of Education at the University of Alberta. As a lifelong learner, Vireo went on to become a facilitator of transformational programs such as Orgasmic Healing, Laughter Yoga, Kundalini Dance™, and Sacred Femininity. She is also trained in mindfulness techniques.

Drawing on her training and education in ways unique to herself, Vireo is an extremely skilled and intuitive facilitator. Using her exceptional knowledge of women's sexuality, a non-judgmental approach, and Belief Re-patterning, she helps her clients to successfully and gracefully transform limiting beliefs so that they can be their best selves. She specializes in shame busting around taboo subjects like sex, grief and suicide.

www.dancingpleasuregoddess.ca /
www. beliefrepatterning.com/team/vireo-karvonen/
https://www.facebook.com/Vireo-Karvonen-Belief-Re-patterning-Life-Coach-2161503237463498

Transforming That Shame

By Vireo Karvonen

I t was May 2016, and I was struggling. I was drowning in my own tears. Some days, I couldn't get out of bed. I was on medical leave. My heart was racing at one, two, three, four, and five in the morning. The many voices in my head were cruel, and oh so loud, screaming at me that I was crazy, stupid, no good. I couldn't silence them. I didn't know how.

This is my story. The story of how, over the following year, I found my own path away from that darkness to a deeper connection with my Self and my inner light by using tools and techniques to achieve deep personal transformation. Prayer, beauty, laughter, dance, and nature became my medicines and granted me access to my intuition. I was also drawn to learn many new practices like mindfulness, Laughter Yoga, ancient sacred sexual healing, and Belief Re-patterning. This is my story of how I came home to my Self and became a shame-buster.

I began to doubt myself while on medical leave the year before. I started to believe that what my own inner critic was saying about me was true. I felt "not good enough" as a teacher. I felt "not good enough" as a mom. I felt "not good enough" as a daughter. My adrenals were stressed, causing adrenaline to pump through my body twenty-four seven. I didn't like myself. I didn't like my life. I felt unlovable. I felt unworthy. I am an educated woman with a master's in education, and yet I couldn't make even the simplest of decisions from one day to the next. At fifty-five years old, I felt like I had wasted much of my life. I felt like I amounted to nothing and I was terrified of being judged by others.

Deep shame began to wrap itself around me, sending me in a downward spiral.

At the end of June 2016, after receiving additional news regarding my mom's ongoing diagnosis with colon cancer, and a letter terminating my teaching contract, I felt I had reached my lowest of low points. The final blow that blew my whole life apart, that broke my heart, came when my beloved partner of three and a half years sent me a text message: "I release you."

I felt completely shattered physically, emotionally, mentally, and spiritually. I felt unworthy of living. I felt needy, powerless, helpless, and pathetic. My life, as I knew it, was completely dismantled. Now I had another failed relationship to add to my list of failures, including my marriage of seventeen years. I began to question and doubt all of my choices in life.

Someone accused me of being a burden to my parents, adding to the shame that was consuming me. Hell, I felt like a burden to myself. I felt ashamed for that neurotic behavior and the destructive thoughts I was having, ever spiraling me down into more shame.

In *Power Vs Force*, David Hawkins says that shame is the lowest vibration on the planet, and we need help to rise above it. I felt my Dad's caring and concern when he took me to the local, small-town hospital. The doctor on duty asked me a myriad of questions: was I planning on killing myself? If yes, how did I plan to kill myself? Within minutes, I walked out the door with a 1-800 number, a prescription, and a tiny Ziploc bag of the antidepressant Celexa (citalopram). I was pissed off at the systems in my life: the public education system and the health care system, which I felt would rather throw a pill at my symptoms than get to the root of the problem. I felt mistreated all round.

Shock and sadness turned into anger, and then rage rose up in me. This turned out to be a blessing in disguise. Hawkins says that, "Anger can lead to either constructive or destructive action."

"Anger can be a fulcrum by which the oppressed are eventually catapulted to freedom. Anger … has created great movements that led to major changes…" (Hawkins, Power vs Force, p. 65).

I felt volatile, dangerous, and out of control, but the energy of anger helped me rise up out of all that shame. Something deep within me, in my body and soul, softly whispered not to take the medication. I had witnessed my older brother Ben's experience with anti-depressants and other drugs for schizophrenia before he took his life. A moment of calmness wrapped itself around me as I tucked the tiny bag of Celexa away and tore up the prescription.

The anger that simmered inside of me fueled my desire to not be medicated and gave me the strength to make three massive life decisions.

First, I chose to close the door on public school teaching for the second and final time in my life. I had taught in the system for a total of fifteen years and it was slowly killing my soul. I quit teaching the first time in 2001 when my second son, Aidan, was born. I had no intention of returning to it. But, the transition from my seventeen-year marriage had led me to my cabin by the lake, where there was no cell reception, no internet, and no reliable income. I chose to put my coaching business on hold because my clients lived two hours away. I was drawn back to the classroom by the necessity of putting food on my table. But this time was different; I left the system for good.

Second, I decided that I would be "sovereign" in my sexuality. I had no idea how, and I didn't even know what "sovereign" meant or where that word came from. I wanted to enter my next relationship from a place of wholeness, especially around my sexuality. I wanted to be able to experience sacred union in my own self pleasuring, making love with myself. I was determined to clear anything that was in the way of my sexual sovereignty.

Third, I decided that I was going to be single for thirteen moons. This meant no dating and no sex with another. Just self-pleasuring. Simply being with myself and coming to deep self-love and wholeness.

My path to freedom was being born. I rode the waves of grief using my Kundalini Dance™ training to help me feel everything and to free myself from the fear, the sadness, the anger, and even the rage. I had been introduced to Leyolah Antara's Kundalini Dance (an ecstatic transformative dance that combines breath, sound, and movement) on my birthday in January 2007. It had been my gift to myself. Kundalini Dance empowered me to come out of the wallpaper and began to shift me from being disconnected to feeling more connected to my body and my Self.

In the summer 2016, I found support and rediscovered the healing power of prayer, forest bathing, the beauty of nature, and animal medicine. As spring rolled into summer, the Alberta wild roses began to draw me out of myself and into life. A festival of colors burst forth, shouting at me to be seen. With my camera, I captured the wild roses at dawn at every stage – birthing buds, unfolding petals, full blooms. Outward beauty called me inward, to a stillness and calm that I hadn't known in a long while.

Nature has the power to reset our brain.

My next lifeline came in the form of dance medicine at a three-day Kundalini Dance retreat on Salt Spring Island. It was on Canada Day weekend, 2016, just days after that shattering week of endings in June. I had messaged Lyndsay, my Kundalini Dance soul sister who was organizing the upcoming workshop, to tell her that I felt too raw and vulnerable to go. She told me then what I tell my Kundalini Dance students and coaching clients now, "that is the reason to come, not the reason not to come." Then she added, "and we will hold you." I wept. Lindsay had been one of the support team members when I took my Kundalini Dance facilitator training back in 2007. I trusted her. A butterfly landed on my body and stayed there for the entire call. The butterfly didn't leave until I said, "Okay, I'll come."

If not for the butterfly medicine that showed up to play with me and whisper gently to me, I might not have said "yes" to that life-changing weekend on Salt Spring island. I danced wildly and passionately, expressing my intentions and my prayers. Snot and sweat were flying everywhere as I let go and began to feel alive and at home in my body again. Cleansing tears flowed as I danced. Courage rose up in me. I felt witnessed and held by my sacred sisters in the dance. Laughter erupted joyously, loudly and unapologetically from my soul as I danced. More tears were loosened, but this time they flowed with a sense of creating space for more joy. I no longer gave a flying fuck what others thought. I felt less alone. I felt connected to myself, to my Self, to Source, to my community of sisterhood. I returned home feeling the beginnings of my liberation. I felt hopeful. I felt more like myself.

As summer turned to autumn, I became a Laughter Yoga Facilitator. I also signed up for an online mindfulness training course, which helped me to be more present in the moment and more connected to simple joys. I began to breathe more deeply and strengthen that thread connecting me to myself. That summer, I walked mindfully barefoot on the grass, and then slowly on the frozen lake as autumn turned to winter. I laughed daily. Instead of adrenaline pumping through my body, endorphins were being released, giving me a natural high.

While on Salt Spring island, I had signed up for Sacred Femininity Training in Thailand. It was January 2017, shortly after my fifty-fifth birthday. Shame silently accompanied me to Thailand. For two decades, I had been studying sexuality and expanding in my own sexual healing, however, when I arrived in Thailand for my Sacred Femininity training with Minke de Vos and Shashi Solluna of Tao Tantric Arts, I quickly felt like I was in kindergarten. I felt humiliated and inadequate. I was shocked to discover that at the age of fifty-five, I still had so much shame trapped in my body and still knew so little about my own feminine body. I felt frustrated and angry that there was so much around my sexuality as a woman that I had never been taught in our western world. Over the seven-week intensive training, the ancient sacred Taoist Tantric practices that I learned, such as how to use a yoni jade egg, supported the transformation of that shame into wholeness. I felt natural and sovereign in my own feminine sexuality. My mindfulness practices helped me to avoid drowning, however I still felt quite raw and extremely vulnerable during the whole experience.

Home again at my cabin by the lake, I continued to practice what I had learned, but I noticed that the more emotional and perhaps spiritual shame persisted. I still felt quite unstable and uprooted in my vulnerability. I had no clue how to deal with all of those unsettling, upsetting emotions and old traumas that were surfacing.

Then, three months later, on June 6, 2017, I attended a Belief Re-patterning® introductory event called, "Inner Critic to Inner Coach." I learned how to transform shame and more. Belief Re-patterning is a seven-step system developed by Suze Casey (www.beliefrepatterning.com) that trains our subconscious mind to go to something uplifting; what Belief Re-patterning practitioners call "the upside," as a habit. This is huge because, ninety percent of the time, our subconscious mind is running the show. Mine had been keeping me stuck for a long time.

At that event, a seed of knowing was planted in both my conscious and subconscious mind. My awareness slowly grew as I began to learn and better understand how my brain works.

I bought Suze Casey's book, *Belief Re-patterning, The Amazing Technique for "Flipping the Switch" to Positive Thoughts* (Hay House, 2012). In the preface, I read that "When I was tired, hungry, or emotionally stressed, I would forget all the enlightened stuff that I knew, and all the doubts, fears, and anger would surface, causing the Inner Critic to take center stage in my life. I had been immobilized by the stories that I was telling myself. I hadn't consciously created my reality." I reread this several times and felt great relief. I realized then that there was nothing wrong with me. I wasn't broken. I wasn't stupid. I wasn't crazy. I simply didn't have access to that part of my brain that would have helped me to make better choices and be my best self. Although I was not consciously aware of it, my Inner Critic, that primal part of my brain, had been dictating my life. Shame stories had been paralyzing me. So, when someone showed up wearing my clothes, acting like a wild, crazy cave woman and behaving in embarrassing, unrealistic ways, I could now have more compassion for her. She was *my* primal wild cave woman.

One month later, I participated in my first Belief Re-patterning signature two-and-a -half day workshop called, "Flip YOUR Switch." Forgiveness for myself gradually emerged as I better recognized that when I was feeling draining emotions like depression, anxiety, profound sadness, heart-breaking grief, lots of upset, and deep hurt, I was operating in my reptilian mind. I could only access what I call the four Fs: fight, flight, freeze, and fuck you. You see, in that state, we do *not* have access to our prefrontal cortex, the rational part of the brain, where uplifting emotions and states of being, like choice, reason, hope, intuition, compassion, kindness, peace, forgiveness, inner peace, and joy, are located. Working with how the brain learns, Belief Re-patterning helps us to navigate from the draining emotions of our Inner Critic, to uplifting emotions by strengthening the voice of our Inner Coach.

At the end of Friday evening, I had a huge moment of extreme panic. I wanted to run very far away from the event and not come back. I could barely breathe, and I was on the verge of tears. I felt so vulnerable, I didn't want to be seen. I approached the door of the conference room with trepidation. One of the women looked into my eyes and I burst into tears. I ran back into the room. Suze Casey, the founder of Belief Re-patterning, came to my side. I was being consumed by shame and fear but didn't know it.

Suze skillfully guided me through her seven-step process of Belief Re-patterning. First, she offered me a drink of water and asked me what word I had chosen from the *Poster of Possibilities* (a poster with 999 words to up your vibration) that evening. My word was "perfection" which initially made no sense to me. Suze muscle tested and asked if there was another word to support me. "Breathe" was my second word. The critical monkey in my mind told her that I couldn't breathe; it was too hard to breathe. Suze then walked me through the Belief Re-patterning seven step system: Forgiveness, Permission, Choice, Freedom, Affirmation, Surrender, and Gratitude.

Suze had me say out loud, "I forgive myself for believing that this panic defines me." She gently guided me to a second forgiveness statement and had me repeat, "I forgive myself for believing that I don't know how to breathe or can't breathe."

Next, we moved to a permission statement, "I give myself permission to dissolve that old panic by breathing." Then Suze suggested some "choice" statements: "I can choose to stay in that panic or I can choose to breathe. I can't do both, so I choose to breathe. I choose to breathe and open to the perfection of my breath."

After I made that statement, I suddenly felt able to breathe. The tears had stopped. Suze and I laughed together. "We're not done yet," she exclaimed, "there are four more steps!" For the next step, she had me create a freedom statement which gave me a specific action to reinforce the feeling. I said, "I am free to breathe deeply and open to the perfection of the moment, when I sit in the hot tub at the pool tonight."

The next step in the process was Affirmation.

Most of the affirmations I had used in the past were unsuccessful because they were about using repetition to convince myself of something that I didn't believe, nor had never experienced as true. Belief Re-patterning uses affirmations to remember a time in the past to tie the current learning to something known that has already been experienced, in this case "perfection" and "knowing how to breathe."

Suze asked me, "When have you breathed and opened to the perfection?" I smiled as I confidently stated, "I know what breathing deeply and opening to perfection feels like, it happened when I was leading root chakra class for Kundalini Dance." I had been leading hundreds of women in Kundalini Dance since 2008. We then claimed the new feelings with "I am opening to the perfection of the moment with my breath"; the Surrender stage. The final Gratitude statement, "I am grateful to myself for remembering to breathe and be open to the perfection of this moment," solidified the re-patterning steps I had taken and reinforced.

In a matter of minutes, I shifted from panic and uncontrollable crying to deep breathing and a new awareness of the perfection of the moment. Belief Re-patterning worked! I found myself again.

Suze noticed that I was reluctant to leave and return to the hotel room that I was sharing with a friend. Another supportive Belief Re-patterning sequence helped me shift from feeling responsible for my brother dying from suicide and the life of a depressed friend (who was sharing my hotel room), to being responsible for my own life. I left, feeling a deep peace and a calmness that I hadn't experienced since the tragic death of my brother Ben in 1992.

The Flip YOUR Switch weekend helped me to start training my subconscious to move toward uplifting positive emotions, "the upside" as a habit. Moving forward from that transformational weekend, I followed Suze Casey's suggestion and began picking a word a day from my *Pocket Full of Possibilities* to guide me toward being more of my best self. That summer, I also said yes to becoming a Belief Re-patterning practitioner, so I could help not only myself, but also others.

I now had a powerful tool to help me navigate my life and transform those shame stories, especially around sexuality, that had been coming to the surface since my training in Thailand. All that shit was now becoming very rich compost for my growth. Over the next many months, I avoided the usual spiralling into old victim stories, draining emotions, and limiting beliefs for days, weeks, months, years, and, sadly, even decades. Instead, I could now access uplifting emotions and more of my best self in seconds, minutes, or, on rare occasions, hours. Freedom! I began using the Belief Re-patterning tool with my coaching clients.

For a long time, shame was the central theme of my life. Today, although some still remains, I no longer lose myself in it. Instead, I now support others by helping them to transform shame and other depleting emotions into life-affirming emotions. Some of my clients have even started calling me "The Shame Buster."

On April Fool's Day (I am not kidding!), my Belief Re-patterning empowered me to give birth to myself as a Sacred Sexuality Coach and launch my online course for women, the *Sacred Pleasure Path Program*. I am a shame buster around all of the taboo subjects: death, suicide, mental health, self-pleasuring, and sexuality. I provide others with powerful tools for rising above shame through my Belief Re-patterning and my Sacred Pleasure Practice.

As women, we are more powerful, confident, and invincible when we are connected, orgasmic, sovereign, and satisfied in our sacred sexuality. The world, in general, fears a sexually empowered woman. However, I have found that it is not the empowered woman who should inspire fear; it is the disempowered woman who is stuck in societal shame and thus behaving irrationally.

Thanks to the transformational power of my personal Belief Re-patterning, I am now grateful for that job ending, for that partner leaving, for that breakdown, and for all that stress because it has all allowed me to come home more deeply to my Self, to be more present in my life, and to feel fulfilled as I inspire other women, their partners, and their families with my soul's work.

As I write this, I hear thunder rolling in the distance. I look across the lake and breathe in the varied shades of green, my eyes wide open, in my full presence and being-ness. I feel so alive. I am so present. The energy of the storm moves through my body and I am turned on.

Just a few years ago, I was unable to be fully present and appreciate the perfection in a moment like this. A tremendous peace and inner tranquility washes over me – my mind, my body, my heart and my soul. I drink up this beauty that surrounds me, that Source has blessed me with. I am feeling whole and at home within myself.

Personal Insights: From Shadows to Light

- I am not alone. You are not alone. Asking for help is brave. Together we can all rise up.
- I am not broken. You are not broken. We all just have old beliefs that have kept us stuck and block our path.
- The power of prayer deepens our faith in something greater than our small selves, and helps us to know that everything is happening *for* us.
- Using Dance as Medicine (Kundalini Dance, Chakra Dance, Qi-Gong) or another conscious movement practice, is very effective in clearing stagnant energy from the body and energy bodies (auric field).
- Nature therapy – forest bathing – has the power to reset our brains. It is important to revel in the beauty of nature every day.
- Walk barefoot on the earth. This will ground you and lower your body's pH.
- Anger can fuel change and action when re-directed consciously.
- Belief Re-patterning transforms guilt, shame, "not enough-ness" to self-acceptance, self-confidence, "enough-ness," and self-love. Belief Re-patterning can also empower us to go from people-pleasing and seeking approval from others to giving our own approval to ourselves.

- Practice mindfulness (mindful walking, mindful breathing).
- Explore how to self-pleasure. Serotonin and oxytocin, natural feel-good endorphins, are released in our bodies when we experience pleasure and healthy touch.
- Laughing every day releases oxytocin and natural, pain-relieving endorphins -like dopamine- into our bodies that give us a natural high. Try Laughter Yoga; you can check mine out on YouTube:
  https://www.youtube.com/watch?v=WCbBjRfy8Qg
- I am a better version of myself because of all my life experiences, including that breakdown and my breakthroughs.
- The more we shine a light on shame, the more it dissolves and no longer has power over us.
- If my story resonates with you, please don't waste another moment of your life. If shame has a hold on you, I encourage you to reach out for support from me or someone in this book who you resonate with. Your liberation and connection await you. You deserve it!
- Your liberation is my liberation. My liberation is your liberation.

Marilyn Brighteyes

Marilyn Brighteyes was born carrying the burden of intergenerational trauma that is the consequence of centuries of colonization in Canada; in particular, the impact that Residential schools had on aboriginal families. She grew up surrounded by abuse, drugs, and 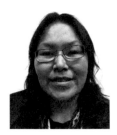 alcohol, but that part of her story is nothing new. What sets her apart, as an individual, is that she has chosen to rise above the trauma. Her mantra is, "It is what it is, until it isn't."

Marilyn is a defiant beacon of truth shining its light on the darkness of genocide and colonization. She has chosen to share her story and shed light on the otherwise taboo subjects of rape and abuse in the family. She has learned that, in order to heal and break the cycle, she must talk about her difficult past and not run from it.

Her kids are her motivation. Today, she takes her journey one step at a time. She has over ten years of sobriety, but she has yet to fully heal from her past and, in truth, still battles her own demons. Along the way, however, she has helped many others talk about their pasts, and heal from their own trauma. She currently works at Boyle Street Community Centre where she is a Support Worker.

http://facebook.com/Cree.made.it

Never Quit, No Matter What

By Marilyn Brighteyes

I am a product of your ignorance. Is that too bold to say? That while Canadians were living off the land of my forefathers, my mom and dad were being beaten and punished for speaking their language. And, while Canadians say "get over it" as they continue to line their pockets with the fruit of stolen lands, our children shed their blood and feed the earth with their lifeless bodies because they have to deal with the repercussions of Residential school and forced assimilation.

As my people grieve their loved ones- lost to addiction, mental health problems and homelessness- most Canadians act like we are invisible, and have the prejudice that we are drunkards and a burden to society. As I watched my brother dig through garbage cans to find enough money to help him forget the rapes he endured in foster care, people pass him by with that judgment.

Day after day, the staff at the Boyle Street Community Services go to work trying to help and give hope to the hopeless, wondering: *Is it enough?* Or will we get the call that says, "I'm so sorry there was nothing more we could have done"? So I ask: when will you wake up and help? When will you be the solution instead of the problem?

This is my story.

My mom survived genocide. Back then, they called it Residential schools or Industrial schools. The children that are my age now have intergenerational trauma, they say. Like so many First Nations, we grew up in addiction and poverty. My mom managed to survive her stay at a Residential school with a quarter of a lung missing and so much trauma that she spent the rest of our lives trying to escape; with alcohol and later on with prescribed drugs. If that wasn't enough, she also had less than a grade six education. She was, however, able to retain her language in spite of the nuns' efforts to crush that out of her. She raised us with a heavy hand that didn't leave room for talking back. As we grew, however, her hardness made us rebel and fight back due to resentments and the loss of our childhood innocence from her drinking and the violence we were surrounded by. Residential school had left many broken homes and were a breeding ground for incest and family violence, to which there didn't seem any escape, except through drugs and alcohol. Yet in our bid for freedom, we ended up becoming everything we ran from. We became the monsters that we fled from.

My mom birthed six children- me being the youngest- yet raised eight off and on. My mom had sold my oldest sister when she was fourteen or fifteen years old. I tell my siblings' stories, as well as my own, because they are interwoven so closely and we were all affected. As a result of this sale, my sister had my niece who was a year and half older than me. My sister's thinking was, since mom was the reason she was raped and impregnated, then she should help raise my niece. So my mom helped look after her. She became my big sister. My nephew also grew up with us off and on. None of my siblings ever really raised their own children. I became the only one able or willing to bring up my kids in this chaotic family dynamic. My earliest memory is of my mom's rape when I was six years old. I remember it so clearly because I was sleeping right beside her when it happened. It was a result of the drinking she did and the men she brought home to pay for her substance use.

As a result of me getting sick shortly after her rape, the four of us ended up in foster care together. At first it was the four of us: my older brother, my niece, me, and my nephew, but then we were separated and I ended up in another home with my brother. We were supposed to be safe in there; however, it was more in the structure of a Residential school. Mistreated and neglected, we lived there for a year and half. My brother later told Mom of our abuse and we were able to go back to her. She sobered up for a bit, but when my cousin tried to rape me when I was nine, my mom gave up- feeling powerless- and went back to her drinking.

Grief. It kills you slowly, knowing that the one you love and need can't be seen or touched anymore. At some point after my cousin's attempt to rape me, my grandma died, which I think also contributed to my mom's drive to drink.

At some point after we moved- we moved a lot as I grew up- I became resentful of my mom's drinking and the continued abuse we endured at the hands of family and friends. We were all back together: my brother, niece, and nephew. My brother became our abuser and Mom was always gone, so we had to learn how to protect ourselves. I was nine when my brother took my virginity and became my living monster that I could never talk about; and, even when I did, it was somehow my fault. After my brother raped me, it became almost normal to be sexualized and abused. I later found it was safer to be amongst strangers because the majority of my abuse was by family. I also found that if you go home with a man, then you can get drunk and fed. I was twelve when I figured that out, so when I turned thirteen my sister confronted me and offered up one of her regulars saying, "It's better than hanging out at the corner." She was looking out for me like big sisters tend to do...

Between the rapes and the prostitution, coupled with my brother's growing anger, I was thirteen when I tried to cut my heart out, hoping that it wouldn't hurt so much if it wasn't there. There didn't seem to be any hope in sight. I was lucky enough to join a drama group after that cutting. From there I began to have hope. I wanted so much to change the life I lived. My oldest sister was the only one that really supported me. I looked up to her in so many ways; she often gave me advice and told me what I shouldn't do. I listened as much as I could. It was difficult being the youngest, though. I struggled with needing to be heard. I was finally listened to in the drama group I had joined. It became my outlet and a place I could share parts of my life and feel validation. It's where the seed was planted that it didn't have to be like this. It was the start of my long journey of cycle-breaking. I did my best to stay in school; however, it's hard to get up in the mornings after taking care of an adult alcoholic. The long nights of keeping Mom and myself safe took their toll.

The man and woman who ran the drama group did their best to help us. Eventually they started a high school for us to combat the effects of childhood trauma and family addictions that prevented us from being able to complete school. In spite of their efforts and guidance, I was unable to complete high school. Instead I became pregnant at the age of seventeen and had my boy at eighteen. I had miscarried at fifteen due to my stepdad's continued rapes. My goal was to be a better parent than my mom was to us. I fought my addictions. Yet, as hard as I tried, my family couldn't or wouldn't let me succeed. We were guilted and reminded of our failings when we tried to get away from addiction. My other older sister was doing the best she could too; however, her dad abused our mom so bad that mom took it out on her. It seemed we were the only two that wanted a different life. My nephew was able to quit as well, after his mother died from her substance use. By then, I could see my family slowly destroying themselves, unable to overcome the trauma of growing up Indian. When I think of this time, I get angry because so many times I heard, "Get over it!", yet First Nations were raised in dysfunction by programs funded by the government. When I met Joe, the man who ran the drama group, he taught me about Residential school. My mom only ever talked about it when she was drunk. I didn't even know until later on that my two oldest sisters had been sent there as well.

After joining the drama group, I could see that this didn't have to be my kids' fate, but I could never visualize anything different. It felt like this is what we were born for, dysfunction and discrimination. Hope was born and then crushed by the reality of life at home. I went to a college and was finally able to graduate, as one of our family's first high school graduates, but I ended up following mom back home to the reserve. A year later, she died. Her lungs having worked for so long with a quarter of one missing, she succumbed to her illnesses. She died from the toxin in her blood that made her lose her mind. She rattled her bed rails. She couldn't be trusted to not walk out of the hospital, so she was tied to her bed; only freed by death, like her eldest children, Peter and Fran. As I write this, one of my older sisters and I are the only ones who have survived out of six of us.

When Mom died, I had just had my fourth child. I dove into depression and my brother was instrumental in keeping me addicted. By the time I had my fifth child, I was ready to quit. I was determined to make a better life for my kids, but this time I was focused on my own self-improvement. I was forced to go to women's groups by child welfare who finally found out about my heavy addictions and stepped in to help change our lives for the better. I started learning about how I was fucking over my kids, and that I was doing the same thing my mom did while raising us. I was determined to not be my mom.

Taking what I learned from the drama group, I went into a training group for group facilitation. It lasted six months: one week on, one week off. I worked on myself and the negative teaching I learned growing up. We used some good authors' teachings and learned to call each other on our bullshit, learned about how to listen and not give advice. I was able to start seeing my patterns of self-destruction and change them. I could self-diagnose because I was shown by the others what to look for. It helps to keep me grounded and out of ego. The women's group that I had been going to as a participant for half a year, was now a group I was able to facilitate. We didn't get paid for it. There was no funding, so we did it for free as well as paid for snacks from our own pockets; something Joe would do for us in the drama group. Things were starting to turn around. I had two years sobriety when I was able to meet my dad again. He had been chased away by Mom when I was around four because he had wanted to take me away to a better life.

My dad, I was told, was Eskimo and from B.C.; that he up and left us, with three hundred dollars' worth of clothes for me. But that was a lie: my dad loved me and wanted to take me with him - away to something better. My mom would tell me his name and make everyone else be quiet and not talk about him. In fact, my dad is a master carver, a hereditary chief of the eagle/beaver clan of the Nisga'a nation, and a recipient of the Order of British Columbia. When he left us, he went back home and learnt his language and culture and made himself great. My youngest daughter looked so much like me that he felt he got me back when she went running into his arms. We moved into his house right away. Like a fairy tale, I was a daughter to a Chief. I was his only living child and I gave him the grandchildren he always wanted. It was short-lived. We moved to Vancouver because I didn't want to go anywhere near my abusive brother. In Vancouver, I was contacted by the daughter of a woman my oldest brother had murdered. She wanted to know his story, but I didn't know it. I told her he had raped me by knife point when I was fourteen, on Christmas Eve. Since we had the same mom, I was able to share my story and the things that made me different from my family. Things like the drama group, the trainings, and the many workshops I was able to go to in order to change my thinking and then change our lives.

We agreed to meet up when I got back home. We eventually did meet, when I moved back to my reserve. I was lucky enough to be involved in another training. This one was focused on addictions, which led to work in a college. Another first, I think. I was lucky to not get caught in my early years; I never had a criminal record, so I was able to get the job. I still didn't know how to drive and no one in my family would teach me.

I learnt from my oldest sister the history of abuse that was in our family. No one talks about it, so nothing is done about it. When my mom charged her nephew for his attempted rape of me, she was cut off. Maybe she was a bitch about it, but what do you expect? When my oldest sister was molested by our uncle when she was seven, my sister was hit by mom and two of our aunties for having told, and then sent to Residential school early. You just don't tell. I learnt about these patterns and heard from many others that share my story. My story is not original. The only difference is that I went against everyone and started sharing what I was raised in.

I started being asked to share my story at various places with the daughter of the woman my brother Peter had brutally murdered years earlier. We met and developed a friendship. We now talk about our story and how we continue to heal from it, together. Forgiveness was the mission that brought us together. You are healed the day you die because you will no longer hurt when you are dead.

The next year, I was given a job at the high school that Joe had started so many years ago. I talked with youth that shared similar stories to mine. I worked through their trauma as we beaded. We used ceremony and an elder to aid in the journey of healing. Hard, but so rewarding.

And then our lives got harder. I always knew that my family would self-destruct eventually. I had thought that it would be me and my nephew that would be the last two standing. I was wrong. He had more sobriety than me, and I was going on ten years. He said, "It's just a number." In fact, he stopped counting at eleven years. But his addictions didn't kill him. He died instantly driving a family back home on Halloween night. Peter and Fran had been the first, and then mom.

Five months later, my oldest sister died the same way mom did. Living on oxygen for a few years, she had still struggled to quit the addiction that killed her. She had one week's sobriety before she died. Later, a few more deaths, and then my boyfriend died. We had just gotten together, and he died of a heart attack. If I hadn't had the years of sobriety that I had, I don't think I could have stayed sober. But I had my kids to think of.

I get asked what keeps me going; what keeps me sober. My answer is, "My kids, the fear of them being abused in a foster home like me, and my family." We were all hurt in the foster care system that was meant to keep us safe- which it didn't- it's a lie people like to tell themselves so they can sleep better at night.

Then, I was laid off, and my son ran away. I held on to hope and my youngest son, grieving the family I could never quite have. I was accepted into this job, working with pregnant mothers who have fallen through the cracks. Women who have lost their other children to the system and are pregnant, homeless, struggling with substance use. We help to stabilize them, take them to appointments, and advocate for them when needed. "Be the change you want to see." I was taught that in one of the many trainings I went to, so I embody it. Nine months into my work, my brother died. And then, the day before his wake, my niece died.

Healing never stops because loss is constant. The hope I have is that eventually my grandkids won't have to struggle with intergenerational trauma and racism, and discrimination will be gone. The only way that can happen is by sharing our stories of pain and triumph, and encouraging people to learn the history of the place they are calling home. To be accountable, but kind, in the sharing of truths.

"Be the change you want to see," means don't just talk about it; *be* it. *Be* the change.

I am still grieving, but I am also triumphant because I am alive to teach my children what living looks like.

I have a vehicle now because an older gentleman that drove me shopping decided to also teach me how to drive on my reserve. I made it on the backs of so many people that helped me get to meetings, school, trainings; so many people who were not family, yet offered me encouragement and praised my accomplishments. The one thing my mom taught me was to never quit.

No matter what!

Personal Insights: From Shadows to Light

- Silence is death. Even if it is hard to speak up, even if people try to shut you up, find a way to share your stories, to bring them to light. It is not the end, but that is where the healing starts.
- Don't be afraid to ask for help if you need it. There are people, groups, and organizations that know where you are coming from and can help you find your way.
- The journey is hard and there are no easy fixes, but it is possible to look forward to a brighter future for yourself, your children, and your community.
- The key to survival is to never quit, no matter what.

Katrina Breau

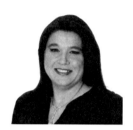 **Katrina Breau** is a Certified Holistic Nutritional Consultant, a brain health and life coach, a guide, and a mentor, who specializes in the use of natural whole foods to promote neurological health, improve cognitive function, decrease health challenges, and build self-confidence.

She draws on her education, her professional experience, and her own personal history of beating the odds, to help people find a workable path to health. Empowering them with attainable short-term goals along the way, she shepherds her clients from a place of isolation and pain to one of joy and balance.

Katrina's passion for helping others live the best and healthiest life possible is obvious to anyone who meets her. Her indomitable spirit and wry sense of humor are always there to remind us that life's challenges are best met with a positive, can-do attitude, even when they appear insurmountable in the moment.

https://www.healthybrain.ca/

Katrina@healthybrain.ca

The Power of Your Shopping Cart

By Katrina Breau

My life's journey has been continuously affected by mental health issues. They have colored every aspect of my life, throughout my childhood, my teenage years, then adulthood. I always felt overwhelmed by the constant change that surrounded me at each stage of my life, and the rollercoaster effect it had on my mental health. By the time I was a teenager, my parents had each divorced multiple times. We were constantly uprooted and moving around to different communities, which meant that my life lacked a solid foundation, and that I had no social network to support me. Adding to that stress, I was also living with the challenges of epilepsy, dyslexia, and sexual abuse. I never felt safe.

Only later in life did I come to understand the impact of this unstable environment on my mental and physical health. The extreme highs and lows of our family dynamic, and the financial consequences of constant change, contributed to a long-term lack of nutritional balance. As a young child growing up with a spectrum of mental and physical health challenges, each meal I ate affected my mood, cognition, seizure activity, and overall wellness. My energy levels fluctuated according to the quantities and qualities of nutritional fuel I received daily. Later, I grew to understand the power of nutrition and how my shopping cart, and the food I chose, could act as a medicine to help my body and my mind be the best it could be.

The rainbow of issues that chipped away at my mental health as a child depleted my self-confidence, which contributed to a lack of self-esteem and self-worth. School was not the exciting opportunity to me as it was for the other children. I always felt humiliated due to my medical condition. In the early 70s, epilepsy was not well understood. My classmates' parents were worried that their children might somehow "catch" this mysterious illness from me or be negatively affected by being near me. The school attempted to relieve the tension by moving my desk to the back of the class. That segregation would become my norm. This added to the lack of cognition and focus caused by the many medications I was on, and it affected me to the point of dysfunction. Even the teachers didn't understand my condition, and, looking back, I don't blame them because, even within the medical field, epilepsy wasn't fully understood yet.

At the age of seven, I was the victim of sexual abuse for the first time. It was at the hands of a twenty-year-old man who babysat me weekly. My parents were not aware of what was happening. I was too afraid to say anything, and my abuser also manipulated me by filling my emptiness with attention.

I was already denied certain foods, such as chocolate, because they increased my seizure potential, but now my diet narrowed even further and the quality of my nutrition deteriorated because my mother could not afford to provide me with regular healthy meals. This negatively impacted my mental health even further.

My personal situation made the already difficult transition to adolescence even more challenging for me. My hormones and medications didn't always agree with each other, causing significant mood fluctuations. I rebelled against the rules of my condition, opting to enjoy sugary treats with the other teens. I would pay for that later. Attending multiple schools in different communities and countries created a lack of social support and provided limited opportunities to develop quality friendships. I was also burdened and overwhelmed with the guilt and shame of being a teenager who couldn't read. I believe that my inability to read came about as a result of being allowed to fall behind in the classroom. Not only was I unable to keep up with the lessons, I was also increasingly isolated from the other students and excluded from classroom activities. My exclusion was compounded by my mother's efforts. She was always pushing me, desperate to prove everyone wrong and desperate to remove the weight of humiliation I carried inside. She would give me the answers to my homework exercises or even do my projects for me. I understand now that she was trying to help me to the best of her ability, but unfortunately, her help only held me back from the educational growth I needed. I don't blame the teachers either because I was never in one school long enough for them to really get to know and understand me or my many struggles.

At home, the cycle of aggression, fear, alcoholism, and all kinds of abuse, continued through the years as my parents went through their various relationships and marriages. I was witness to this turmoil, watching the situation escalate and spill over into my own emotional brokenness. I was often put in the middle of situations that no child or teen should have to deal with. These stressors further worsened my epilepsy, as my seizures were often triggered by high levels of stress. The fear of going home from school was a challenge I dealt with daily. What would the environment be like when I opened the door? Had the alcohol already ignited friction? Sometimes I would stay over at neighbors' homes to feel safe. My neighbors and the teachers at school saw this behavior as a red flag, along with any increase in mood or behavioral changes, which tended to correlate with an increase in seizure activity. It wasn't long before social services removed me from my mother's home and placed me in the foster care system.

I was placed with a very encouraging couple who supported me with each challenge I encountered. They also provided quality food, introducing much-needed nutritional balance into my life. They arranged to have a private teacher come to the house to bring my educational level up from early elementary to where I needed it to be to fit in with my age group at school. I finally started to feel safe enough to grow and develop into the person I was meant to be.

As I began to feel my confidence build, I embraced my new learning and potential, sharing it by tutoring others that faced similar challenges. I took on many jobs in our community as a church youth leader and as a community support worker for special needs children. This work made me realize that no matter how broken I was, there was always someone who had a greater need than I did. I had the ability and opportunity to positively impact them in the way my various neighbors had done for me throughout the years. Looking back, I was so grateful for the warmth those neighbors brought to my childhood. Now it was my turn to uplift others, and I loved the way their faces would change when they realized that someone cared.

While I was helping others, I was always working on myself, finding growth opportunities to keep my momentum going. I discovered a teen community Al-Anon group, where learning the twelve-step program helped me understand my parents' brokenness. The cadet program provided me with a chance to discover my leadership and teaching skills. My epilepsy prevented me from getting a driver's licence at sixteen, but I didn't let it hold me back. Biking was my means of transportation and my chance to enjoy nature. My confidence continued to grow.

Heading into my later teen years, I felt like I was on a mission to prove my past critics wrong. Although I kept up my growth and momentum, I did hit some unexpected brick walls along the way.

One incident that was particularly hard for me to recover from, one that left me in fear for years, was yet another rape: I was raped again by an adult authority figure. As a young child, I thought that I had done a good job of stuffing away the emotional pain of my rape at seven years old; this time, the experience was much more impactful. To make it worse, I became pregnant, and chose to have an abortion, which had me swirling down the drain of depression. I didn't know if I could make it out. Suicidal thoughts overwhelmed me daily. How could I be a leader with this additional humiliation and shame? I was failing to meet the expectations I had for myself, my foster parents, and society's expectation of young girls. I became very introverted as I tried to rebuild my self-esteem.

A year or so later, my drive to overcome the depression and trauma returned with a vengeance. My mission had been reset; lit by a new fire to succeed. This was my life and I was in control of it. I knew I could get back up, brush myself off, and step out of the shell I had built around myself for protection. Returning to become an active member of society once again, I took on many jobs to create a protective, financial cushion around myself, allowing me the opportunity to embrace whatever path I wanted for my life. I was in my final year of high school and the opportunities were endless.

At eighteen, emotionally and financially stable, I started to work in the field of physiotherapy as an aide, assisting with physically challenged children during the day. I took on additional evening and weekend jobs including clearing land, chopping wood, painting houses, and childcare provider to build my financial foundation for my post-secondary education. But within the next year, my plans changed again.

I found myself at a different crossroads: I had been asked for my hand in marriage. My fiancé was older than me, but with all of my life experience, I didn't really relate well to guys my age. Despite the age difference, we had a special bond. We shared similar journeys, both soaked in alcoholism and family trauma.

My husband and I have now been married for over thirty years. We have been through some difficult times, but that has only made us stronger. Soon after we got married, we were relocated to Germany through his job in the military, and I became pregnant with our first child while living on the military base. The doctors on the base didn't think that an epileptic should be having a child; my medication could harm the baby. They advised against this risk and suggested that I abort, but I chose to continue, understanding the risks. Despite some complications during my pregnancy, I gave birth to a healthy child.

As a married couple, we faced many painful mental health challenges, which we overcame together. My husband's alcoholism affected his health, career, our relationship, and our children. Although the experience was very painful, he was able to escape the magnetism of this addiction, surrounded by our love. I supported our family with the assistance of our church and the Twelve Steps to Emotional Healing program. This was a time of extreme stress, not only with respect to my husbands' journey, but also my own. I found myself stuck on the fast-paced rush of society's expectations. I was trying to do it all: as a professional, as a supermom, and as a community volunteer. Life was a mad rush: rushing to daycare and work in the morning, rushing to collect the kids from daycare, rushing to eat, rushing through our evening activities, and then falling into bed, only to do it all again the next morning.

Traveling through life at warp speed, I was in the car a lot, driving throughout the day. As luck would have it, through no fault of my own, I was in many car accidents, which caused some of my neurological challenges to resurface. After I had worked so hard to establish myself in my career, I found myself on disability. I was angry; why did this have to happen to me? Why at a time when I was doing so well? When I was managing to juggle everything so effectively? Or, so I thought.

In the midst of my recovery pity party, my then three-year-old son came to me, shining the light on my brokenness as he patted my hand and said in a way only a three-year-old can, "I'm so glad you are home with us now, Mommy." It broke my heart that it took the seriousness of an accident for me to see that my children missed me. This reality check led me to shift my priorities. I decided not to return to work, but to step into the role of a stay-at-home, full-time wife and mother instead. I was still an over-achiever; I felt it wasn't enough to just be any mom on the block: I had to be Super-Mom.

I made my kids' lives so busy that I transferred my stress onto them. I became so involved in their school and activities that my stress levels came close to reaching what they had been during my corporate years. My last car accident also contributed to an increase in the frequency of my seizures, which led to the loss of my driver's license. Being prohibited from driving greatly impacted my Super-Mom persona and my ability to say yes to all extra activities and commitments. I was suddenly dependent on others to shuttle my kids and me to school and other activities. It was during this period that I became aware of a victim mentality that had been ingrained in me by the trauma of my childhood. Swirling down the drain of depression again, I became sullen and withdrawn.

What led me out of the darkness was my volunteer work with St. John Ambulance, along with the support leader positions I held at our church. I transitioned from volunteering, to casual, to full-time employment as an instructor. My services were in high demand, and it was as an instructor that I discovered a deep passion for both teaching and bringing safety to every household. Both my children also joined in volunteering with St. John Ambulance, and we became a small army of do-gooders. At this time, I was also taking courses in the field of health care. After another decade, I shifted my focus from full-time instructor to full-time caregiver in mental health homecare, in geriatric/palliative facilities, and in hospital settings. The work was rewarding and satisfying, but I was over-stressed due to cutbacks and increased demands on my time. I was heading for another burn-out. Switching to shift work allowed me to homeschool our children during the day and work at night. I thought that this would give our family more quality time together. Not surprisingly, the demands of my work quickly squashed that idea. The love I had for my role as a caregiver led to me to volunteer to take on double shifts. This allowed my coworkers with younger families to spend more time at home with their toddlers, while I covered staff shortages. As the years went by, I continued to routinely work 16 to 18-hour shifts. I not only felt obligated to provide great care to the residents and support for my colleagues, but I was also motivated by the fact that my children were entering post-secondary and those expenses were looming.

After years on that hamster wheel of a career, I put my health in jeopardy to the point of life-threatening vulnerability. I wasn't getting proper nutrition, or sleep, or taking care of my mental health. The stress on my system affected me mentally, emotionally, and physically. It finally culminated in triggering a serious tonic-clonic seizure during which I lost consciousness and experienced oxygen deprivation to the brain and body, along with many other complications. Luckily my husband and son were home to deal with the 911 situation in time. The severity, long-term side effects, and cognitive decline that followed finally created a desire in me to make a permanent change. The mirror I held up to myself reflected all the truths I couldn't previously see, and that clarity led to an epiphany that changed my life.

I realized that my situation would only get worse if I kept going as I had been. With this new perspective and a sense of urgency, I refocused my efforts on transforming myself. I shifted my studies to nutrition, brain health, and life coaching. I not only desperately needed tools from these fields to improve my life, but I felt a calling to share the positive, impactful life lessons I had learned with others. Each course brought up more questions inside of me and a desire to find the answers. My whole body and life changed when I started to put myself first. Now that I was no longer focused on the demands of work, I could enjoy the benefits of every area of my life. I made changes and room for personal spiritual growth, creativity, joy, social pursuits, genuine relationships, relaxation, home cooking, physical activity, and, most importantly, positive brain health. Having cared for people with brain health conditions within geriatric and palliative health care environments, I understood the link between brain health and quality of life. I had often witnessed people who had worked hard to fund a quality retirement, but were unable to enjoy it due to their premature physical or mental decline. I knew I couldn't allow this to happen to me. My stress, depression, and epilepsy could all be contributing factors that would increase my health risks now and down the road.

I knew that, in particular, I needed to significantly change my approach to life and nutrition. It was time to switch directions for a new adventure where I was in full control with the power of *now*. I started educating myself about the effects different foods have on our bodies. Research increasingly confirms that food is medicine. My desire to find answers for myself led me to get certified as a holistic nutritional consultant, a brain health coach, and a life coach. With tools acquired in the process, I'm now helping others improve their lives through nutrition, just as I had.

With the assistance of nutrition, I started to release the mental burdens that came from layers of past pain and were contributing to my daily mood. I made positive changes to my shopping cart, knowing that the power to aid (or hinder) my brain health was within reach. My healthier food choices helped to reduce the impact of depression, anxiety, chronic stress, brain fog, and memory loss, for me as well as my family. I used the experimental method to improve my meal choices and I learned how to use nutrition to alleviate many symptoms of my brain health conditions.

Take simply drinking more water, for example. Increasing water intake has been shown to increase blood flow and oxygen throughout the brain, decrease headaches, and reduce stress effects, while supporting the flow of nutrients throughout the whole body. Drinking more water helped to improve my concentration and cognition, balance my mood and emotions, and improve my slipping memory.

Poor diet and stress have been found to be a major cause of inflammation, which can lead to depression and dementia. I realized that I had experienced more than my share of depression symptoms and high stress throughout my life already; I didn't wish to contribute to the potential of my dementia-directed path any longer. I learned to implement better nutrition so I could create a protective path for my future. Omega-3 fatty acids found in fish have been proven to aid in decreasing destructive inflammation. Choosing to eat more cold-water fish (salmon, herring) helped me to stabilize my moods and diminish my depressive feelings. My active choice to enhance my brain's balance by increasing healthy proteins and good fats with each meal helped me to feel more optimistic, enthusiastic, calm, and compliant. I also started eating a lot more greens. High-quality fruits and veggies are high in antioxidants and provide a potent energy reward. I started eating a whole rainbow of fruits and veggies daily, which gave me the spark I needed to be highly functioning every day.

These days, we keep hearing that more children are suffering from psychiatric disorders. More people are also suffering from anxiety and are in greater danger of having their retirements stolen by Alzheimer's disease or dementia. But what are we to do as individuals to maintain our physical and mental health? If you put diesel into a gasoline-driven car, it will seize up. So why do we keep putting the wrong fuel into our precious bodies? Our grocery carts are where our fuel choices occur. While shopping, most people like myself are always thinking breakfast, lunch, supper, snacks, rather than considering the symptoms of their family members and researching what foods are required to offset and decrease their symptoms. But imagine what could happen if we all just took on a new mindset; one focused on discovering what our systems and bodies truly needed as quality fuel?

In his book *Feel Better Fast and Make it Last,* famous psychiatrist Dr. Aman advises us all to tell ourselves, "When I am tempted by French fries, sugary treats or soda, I will resist and say to myself, 'I only love foods that love me back.'" Let's take action now to fill our carts with the foods that will love us and our family back. Let's use our carts to increase our family's brain health and mood, one meal at a time.

Some families are impacted by budget and can't afford quality foods, or so they believe. In 2018, a major Canadian food study showed that the proportion of food-insecure adults that had received treatment in the previous year for conditions that included anxiety, depression, mood disorders, and suicidal thoughts, was more than double that of adults who had had an adequate amount of food to eat. Food insecurity is a drain on our mental health resources. To combat this epidemic, there are many programs within our Canadian communities that help raise the quality of food and nutrition coming into homes. Your choice in food quality and quantity can be improved by simply joining and getting involved in any of the many community kitchens and food co-ops across Canada. You will be amazed at the benefits and friendships that come out of helping each other.

This has become a new area of focus for my family. I wanted our children to truly understand the realities of food insecurity, and to see how the small choices we make can contribute to positive changes. Not only changes on our table, but on the tables of everyone in our community. We had times when we were supporting our family of four on a very limited income, but we still needed to make food improvement choices. We managed to do it by making use of the opportunities available within our community, church kitchen programs, discount bread basket stores, marked down groceries, and the *Food for Good* programs. We also volunteered our time to aid the causes when finances were tight, contributing at soup kitchens and delivering food hampers. Years later, when we had more of a financial cushion, we continued to donate our time as a family, so our children would always understand the delicate balance of necessity.

My lifelong struggles with the effects of food and nutrition on my physical and mental health have taught me many important lessons that I implement today when I help others see the truth in their food stories. Now that I have clarity regarding the many links between food and overall health, I have found both my true

"Why" and the motivation to walk alongside others as they discover the power of food.

Next time you step into the grocery store, consider your family's health needs or challenges and look at the content of your grocery aisles as medicine for your body. By choosing foods that will love your family back, you will be choosing to level out mood swings, increase energy, improve brain function, improve self-esteem, and build harmony in your home. Embrace the power of your shopping cart and remember you can change, starting now!

Personal Insights: From Shadows to Light

- We are in control of our own destiny, no matter how broken the foundation.
- We have the power and freedom of choice.
- We can all reinvent our life's journey starting today. That imaginary ideal life we all have in our minds can become a vision for real change.
- Our food choices may help create the right chemistry in our bodies for internal healing.
- A higher water intake can have amazing health benefits.
- Eating lots of wild fish and shellfish can also have wonderful benefits. For example, shrimp boosts choline, which helps the brain make acetylcholine, which in turn is very important for memory and cognition. For me, adding protein to a meal is a way of investing in my own brain health with every bite.
- I recommend painting a fruit and vegetable rainbow in your shopping cart every time. High-quality antioxidant produce like blueberries, blackberries, cranberries,

strawberries, raspberries, red and purple grapes, cherries, spinach, Brussel sprouts, broccoli, beets, and red bell peppers, add color, taste and creativity to each meal.

- Unless you have a specific allergy or other medical reason for avoiding any of them, I suggest eating more avocados, nuts and seeds, olive oil, medium chain triglycerides (MCT), coconut oil, green tea, garlic, turmeric, and ginger. They are all great choices to keep our brain and body functioning optimally throughout the day.
- Keep frozen, organic, squeezable baby food blends of fruits and veggies in your car or bag as a healthy alternative to fast-food or a chocolate bar. In my experience they are an amazing option, and my kids loved them.

Ruthann Weeks

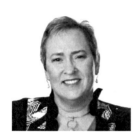

Ruthann Weeks is the founder of Harmony in the Workplace. She is a tireless forward-thinking crusader whose efforts have helped to bring the importance of an abuse-free work environment to the forefront of public awareness. She is also a gifted corporate keynote speaker who delivers a powerful message about today's workplace challenges to senior executives and decision makers.

Starting off as a Certified Information and Referral Specialist in the human service sector, Ruthann went on to graduate as a Human Resource Manager. She also obtained her Canadian Mental Health Association (CMHA) certification as a Psychological Health and Safety Advisor.

Ruthann discovered that the more she learned about workplace bullying, sexual harassment, and psychological safety, the more she wanted to improve the workplace environment for everyone. She established her social enterprise to foster safety in the workplace by addressing violence and harassment through practical education and risk-mitigating strategies. Ruthann donates a portion of all revenues to domestic violence prevention initiatives.

https://www.harmonyintheworkplace.com
https://www.facebook.com/HarmonyInTheWorkplace/
https://www.linkedin.com/in/ruthann-weeks-14650b7b/

Take the Helm

By Ruthann Weeks

I am a natural born planner. It's just the way I'm hardwired. I can't *not* look to the future. You say, control freak; I say, visionary. I like to know what's coming my way, to foresee the changing tides and currents so I can be prepared to navigate the waters of life. The problem with that is, much like real waterways, life is unpredictable.

In my early thirties, I became quite sick. Although I trivialized it, my quality of life was greatly affected, and because of my illness, I could not travel any significant distance without making frequent stops. Even though I was in a serious relationship, I suffered in silence because I was too ashamed to tell my partner what was going on with me. I didn't have a name for the illness at the time and I didn't understand how serious it was. I didn't seek medical attention because I just didn't want to "go there." I hoped it would go away on its own, as mysteriously and swiftly as it had come about.

The disease, I found out later, was Ulcerative Colitis. It is a bowel disease that is incurable, except by surgically removing the affected section of colon. I didn't know why I was sick but then I learned that, while the causes of autoimmune diseases are not fully understood, there is a strong correlation with stress. That explained it. I was going through an incredibly stressful time in my life. My partner was healing from a serious motorcycle accident. He was nearing the end of his disability benefits and had no plans for a new career now that he was unable to work as a mechanic. I'd been laid off from my job, and we were preparing to move across Canada to pursue new possibilities.

While most of the time I kept my cool on the outside, there was no fooling my body; inside, I was experiencing extreme unease and anxiety. Moving away from the only home I'd ever known and sailing toward an uncertain future four thousand kilometers away, took a considerable toll on my body. Out loud, my mouth said all the right things: "I have faith that everything will work out," "At least we have each other," "There are many more opportunities for employment and prosperity out west." My body, however, was privy to my inner dialogue. The fear, angst, and turmoil I was experiencing showed up in my guts.

I was too stubborn and embarrassed to admit the problem to anybody, including myself. Sick as I was, we left New Brunswick and headed across the country with our beloved German Shepherd and our two cats in an old Chevy, hauling a six-by-twelve-foot U-Haul that contained all of our worldly possessions. All we had was four thousand dollars to cross the country and set up a new life in Edmonton. We were fortunate to have friends and family to stay with while we got settled and looked for work. I was blessed to find a job in business administration right away, but my partner struggled to find gainful employment. He had still not recovered physically from his accident and there were limited opportunities that suited his competencies. Money was tight. We still had a home for sale back east and our debt was mounting. My physical symptoms continued to worsen; I finally went to see my family doctor.

My condition was serious enough that I got in to see a gastroenterologist the day after making the decision to get help. I was scoped and, fortunately, there were no tumors, but I had sixty centimeters of ulcerated colon. We started a series of treatments that included steroids and powerful immune blocking drugs. Nothing helped to stop the symptoms. On the contrary, the disease seemed to respond by throwing a temper tantrum, as the symptoms moved from my colon to my joints and limbs. My illness intensified. I developed joint pain and experienced golf ball-sized lumps in my legs. My condition just got worse and worse, to the point that we were considering surgery, which would mean a colostomy bag and a long recovery. But then I experienced a major mental shift that started my journey to wellness.

I had come to the end of myself. I experienced the painful but necessary awakening that I needed to move forward in my life. I heard a message in my faith community that resonated with me and revealed how I would be able to gain my freedom: freedom from stress, freedom from struggle and worry, and, ultimately, freedom from the severity of my illness. I acknowledged my broken, starved spirit and surrendered my life, in its entirety, to a power higher than myself. The strong-willed control-freak in me broke. It was the pivot point that led to an incredible journey of self-discovery and purpose.

Once I surrendered my perceived control, my health started to improve. Slowly and steadily, I was able to maintain wellness using only anti-inflammatory medication and abandoning the powerful drugs that were damaging my liver. It was only when I made the connection between what was happening in my head and what was manifesting in my body that I recognized any responsibility for my illness. I realized that my mental health is largely responsible for my physical condition as it relates to this disease. I now engage in a regular routine of self-care that involves spiritual, physical, and mental health practices. I am diligent about walking outside at least forty-five minutes on most days and paying attention to my natural surroundings. I watch my diet and include lots of fruits and vegetables. Most important, is the time I spend in prayer and meditation. I write out scripture and journal prayers. I find it encouraging to go back and read through my writing and see how things have worked out. This is critical for the over-thinking, future-focused planner in me.

Our minds are so very powerful. Our thoughts are either leading us towards peace and healing, or into fear and anxiety. We have the opportunity every minute of every day to think, feel, and choose our actions with our free will. It's not always easy to choose the positive, and sometimes we need a period of time to feel the pain and angst, but we do not have to drop anchor there. Choosing hope and gratitude, even in our mess, has a profound affect on our brain chemistry and mental health.

***

Despite vast improvements in my mental and physical health, my ulcerative colitis can flare up at any time. One such time was four years ago in connection with a toxic workplace environment. I was working in the non-profit sector as a Certified Information and Referral Specialist. I had just left a long-term job I loved but no longer found challenging, to accept a position as a director with a larger non-profit organization. Becoming a department head was the natural next step in my career path; unfortunately, the new position was a bad fit from the start, and I struggled to find my place on the leadership team. After three months of poor communication and mismanagement, I was let go without good cause and without any opportunity to defend myself.

I was devastated but also relieved. I knew that I was not a good fit with the authoritative leadership style of the organization and my body knew it too. Working there was not good for my health. I would start off relatively fine early in the day but, by the afternoon, I would experience severe flare-ups of my colitis symptoms. I was fatigued from blood loss and lack of sleep, and I was mentally drained as I tried to think my way out of the toxic situation. Relieved as I was to be out of that unhealthy environment, my shiny new opportunity for career growth had evaporated, and I was lost, wounded, and, quite frankly, pissed off. I was left with an empty slate. No plan in sight and no career prospects in an economic recession. Not a comfortable place for anyone, but especially uncomfortable for a planner like me.

It was at that time that God tapped me on the shoulder and reminded me that I'd always wanted to work for myself. My recent experience with unfair treatment in the workplace had opened my eyes to a need that was not being addressed in the industry: workplace bullying. When I was in the situation, I didn't recognize it for what it was, but as I read and learned more about the various types of bullying behaviours, I realized that I had experienced a textbook example of covert bullying tactics. I knew that I was struggling to fit in, but I had no idea that my character was being defamed and disparaged behind closed doors. I was feeling deeply wounded, but learning that what I had experienced was bullying at least validated the shame and devastation I was feeling.

Although there was a growing awareness of violence and harassment in the workplace, I realized that other people suffering in abusive workplace environments might still not know how to recognize and name what was happening to them. After doing some preliminary research and focused soul-searching, I founded my business Harmony in the Workplace to address toxic workplace culture.

I'd like to say that I hit the ground running and that my business was immediately successful, but it was not the case. I was still hurt, and I spent that Canadian winter engaging in rudimentary self-care: taking a lot of bubble baths, binge watching Netflix, and eating too much comfort food. I was fortunate in that I did not succumb to despair for prolonged periods. I asked my doctor if I was depressed. She asked me if I ever felt "down" for a solid two weeks or more. Fortunately, my dark and down periods usually lasted only two or three days and then I would rebound into some semblance of organized optimism. My doctor concluded that I was not suffering from depression.

One of the ways I was able to stay out of the pit of despair was by immersing myself in service to others. There is a coffee shop in a town near me that operates largely on volunteerism and donates tips and profits to community initiatives that support people in practical ways. I started volunteering there once a week for a four-hour shift. I was searching for purpose and belonging. I found it there. I've heard it said that the best way to get out of your own mess is to seek opportunities to serve. For me, this proved to be true. Those caring and spiritual ladies at the coffee shop helped me far more than I ever helped them by making sandwiches and lattes. I continued to volunteer there for two years while I worked on healing myself and growing my business.

***

The more I read, studied, and learned about workplace bullying, sexual harassment, and domestic violence, as well as psychological health and safety, the more passionate I became about bringing awareness and prevention strategies to business and industry, where workplace safety is a constant concern. I felt that I had finally found the challenge I'd been craving and that I knew my purpose: to help create safety for employees in abusive, unhealthy work environments, while teaching employers how to be supportive and meet their legal obligations. So many people were suffering mentally, emotionally, and physically, just like I had; now I could use my gifts to help them. As a Human Resource Specialist, I wrote a training program that covers the legal framework that defines the various types of workplace abuses; establishes expected and prohibited conduct; shows how to develop risk-mitigating policies and responsive procedures; shows how to build a case if you are experiencing workplace abuse, and outlines how to respond and investigate allegations as an employer. It is important to me that employers know how to create healthy and productive work environments and that workers know their rights and are empowered to act when they see or experience abuse.

In the past, I worked as an information and referral specialist for many years at a non-profit resource center. I was privileged to assist people in crisis, to hear their stories when they were at their most vulnerable and help them devise plans to access resources

138

that addressed their issues. They often did not seek assistance until they were feeling helpless and hopeless. The issues they faced frequently involved financial crisis and a lack of knowledge about available programs and support. Sometimes it was a senior needing help with snow shoveling or transportation to medical appointments, or a parent seeking support and encouragement for dealing with their drug-addicted teen. The most rewarding part for me was to see their stress levels drop as they gained hope and found light in their hardship. Leaving my office with a plan, knowing that I was going to follow up with them, both empowered them and left them feeling less isolated in their struggles.

Life is messy. Every one of us will face circumstances bigger than ourselves at some point; something larger than the work we do or the hats we wear as boss, employee, parent, son/daughter, friend. It might be a divorce, a death, a job loss, a health or mental health crisis, or it might be a toxic relationship that reduces us down to our raw selves. We all deserve grace and dignity in our mess, even at work. In safe, healthy, and supportive workplace environments, it's okay to not be okay. The time I spent in client services gave me valuable insight and great empathy for people. That insight, coupled with my human resource management training and education, now positions me to better serve employers by helping them support their workers and transform their organizations.

One of the areas in which I'm passionate about creating change is workplace *psychological* safety. Psychological safety is about trust. We all need trust at work. We trust that our colleagues are going to show up for work, we trust that our clients are going to pay us, we trust that we are going to get our vacation time and promised benefits. Psychological safety is a level above that trust. It takes into account workload management, civility and respect, recognition and reward, and other factors that contribute to an organizational culture where is it safe -even encouraged- to speak up. It was a lack of psychological safety that led to me being pushed out by my workplace bully. I was not free to ask questions or express ideas. I was perceived as threatening and as someone who didn't "fit in."

In a psychologically safe environment, expressing ideas, and reporting mistakes and near misses is encouraged. Without fear of reprisal, issues can be addressed openly and corrections can be made. Organizations that embrace psychological safety consistently build effective teams and efficiencies; they are always improving and fostering innovation. They become the employers of choice where engagement is high and business thrives.

Savvy employers recognize that we are in a social shift, and that the *status quo* is no longer enough to attract and retain top talent. Key personnel aren't protected simply by their performance numbers but are evaluated on their interpersonal skills as well. In an increasingly competitive environment, social attributes such as civility, respect, and teamwork are now showing up on reviews and factoring into promotions and salary increases.

I have been given a big vision and I have big goals. I have been told by wise men that I would not have been given a vision that I would not be fully resourced to see through. I believe them. I run my business as a social enterprise that exists to bring understanding and preventative measures to toxic workplace cultures that cause people to suffer in unhealthy environments. I not only work to get leadership on board, but increasingly deal directly with employees, especially where management is not responsive to their concerns. My vision is that we will create harmonious workplaces where people treat each other with civility and respect, where there is grace enough for someone to have a bad day, and where there is no fear of reprisal for standing up to an abusive boss or workplace bully. I look forward to the day when mental health challenges are understood; where it's okay to not be okay; where there is a shared corporate vision that creates a cohesive team working toward a common goal; where colleagues share in the business of life, the celebrations, and the heartaches too. A workplace where harmony reigns.

***

I can joyfully report, with much gratitude, that I have not had a colitis flare up in three years. Does this mean that I've not experienced stress during that time? No, quite the contrary. I am in the process of building a business, while raising a teenager, and assisting my aging parents. What I can say, is that I'm walking in my power and my light. I have found great freedom in agreeing to not know all the details about where I'm headed and how I am to get there. Instead, I rest in the knowledge that whatever the future has in store for me, it will be good, and that I am loved and cared for. I believe that my future is bright.

Although my personal experiences have been painful and humbling, I would not change a thing because they have all led me to the discovery of my purpose. Every day I learn more about how powerful our thoughts are, how we can create future memories and choose where we are going for ourselves. Whatever our current circumstances, we can choose to become the people we want to be simply by deciding to focus our minds on what we can do and accomplish. I have discovered that we don't have to know the details of how we are going to reach our destination; what a relief! We simply must agree to follow our path when it becomes known to us, as we continue to walk in our truth with integrity and faith.

I believe that when it comes right down to it, it is hope that gives people the strength to carry on. Faith is the belief that what we hope for will come about. We can't always find it within ourselves. Our human strength is too fragile to consistently overcome the pressures of life. We need a support system of caring individuals in our lives that we can count on, but even they, in their well-intentioned humanness, fall short. I have found that it is only by looking at the bigger picture that we see that our overwhelming problems are suddenly small and insignificant. When we surrender as spiritual beings created for a specific purpose and we seek to walk in divine power to fulfill that purpose, the possibilities become boundless, far beyond what we could imagine for ourselves.

When I am feeling overwhelmed, under-resourced, or scattered, I acknowledge my feelings and practice self-care. I take mental health breaks in the middle of my workday when I am feeling bogged down. I usually go for a walk with my dog (I'm of the mind that all dogs are therapy dogs!) Sometimes I drink a cup of tea or have a glass of wine with a trusted friend. Other times it is as simple as a bubble bath to relax and unwind. I know I am too precious to be left behind and that the Creator has not brought me this far to see me fall. I know there is a purpose to what I experience in life, including my pain and struggles. I give myself permission to be vulnerable. I seek opportunities to serve in ways that will fill my cup. I create a future memory of the person I want to be in my wildest dreams and start intentionally living as that person. Every day, I make the choices that person would make.

As we navigate the waters of life, we need to seek wisdom and discernment in the choices we make every day. I don't always get it right. I am not always kind to myself and I often still find myself trying to walk in my own power. Maybe I'm a slow learner. Regardless, I surrender. Again, and again, and again. I remind myself to be gentle with myself and to speak in my inner dialogue as I would to a dearly loved friend. I forgive myself and carry on walking, not in my own power but in the power of the Creator. A dearly loved child of God, resting in mind, body, spirit, and soul in His intimate love and empowerment. I make the choice every day to walk in the light; to embrace my gifts and purpose; to do the best I can to create change in my section of the pond.

"For I know the plans I have for you," says the Lord. "They are plans for good and not for disaster, to give you a future and a hope." ~ Jeremiah 29:11

Personal Insights: From Shadows to Light

- The only thing I have any control over is me. When I get all caught up in worry or strife over things I can't control, I am wasting my good energy.

- I am a spiritual being with a physical body. Feeding my spirit with what fills my cup is what brings value and richness to my life.

- Simple doesn't mean easy. It is a very simple but difficult thing to surrender control of my life to a higher power.

- Life's greatest gift is to know your purpose. I am blessed to know my purpose and passion.

- All dogs are therapy dogs (cats are ok too – don't tell the dogs!) Animals are so therapeutic!

- Nature is a profound aspect of nurture. Nothing compares with fresh air and sunshine to recharge and refresh.

- That person you think has it all together? They don't. Don't compare yourself to anyone else. Comparison steals joy. Better to concentrate on being your best self.

- When we dwell on our mess, we attract more mess.

- Gratitude is freedom. By consciously re-directing our thoughts towards gratitude, we can shift our energy and mood. Being grateful in every circumstance is freedom from being negatively reactionary.

- By envisioning ourselves living our ideal life, we can create our future.

- We can overcome our subconscious programming. We can challenge limiting beliefs and judgments and consciously change them over time.

- God is *for* us. Discovering that I am a dearly loved child, created for a specific purpose, and with divine power and inspiration, is really what it's been all about for me.

- We experience incredible spiritual power when we are open. Divine power and inspiration are infinite and earth-shaking.

- We must forgive ourselves, often. I mess up daily and tend to beat myself up over it. I need to allow myself the grace to not be perfect, and to be gentle with myself.

- Learn to speak to yourself the same way you would to a beloved friend.

- Grace starts with me; with each and every one of us.

- If we expect patience and forgiveness from others, we must be prepared to forgive others.

- Every day we choose how to be in the world. Choose to be kind.

Olivia Kachman

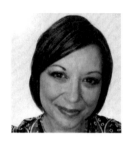 **Olivia Kachman**, B. Ed., discovered her life purpose as a sacred witness who empowers others to heal their lives from the inside out. As founder of Phoenix Alchemy, Olivia is a Transformational Guide, here to serve those who are ready to rise up and feel the freedom of living their fullest potential; a life beyond their past wounds.

Olivia creates a safe, sacred space and intuitively guides people to let go of their limitations and suffering, so they can reclaim their power and rebirth themselves anew. Her offerings include individual and group healing ceremonies, transformational energy work, spiritual dance and embodiment practices.

She honors her teachers, ancestors and spirit guides who continue to awaken the 'medicine woman' within her soul. Olivia is blessed to be a student of Leyolah Antara, a priestess from the Rose Mystica tradition, who initiated her in the lineage of Kundalini Dance™ as a facilitator in 2011. In addition, she owes so much of her own self- empowerment to the 8th Fire teachings of Pete Bernard- a fifth generation medicine man from the Algonquins of Pikwàkanagàn First Nation in Golden Lake, Ontario, Canada.

Olivia's medicine name, Fire Phoenix Dancer, continues to inspire her to follow her calling of helping others to "dance through the flames of transformation" with grace.

Connect with Olivia Kachman

Compiler of *From Shadows to Ligh*t: *A Whole Human Approach to Mental Health.*

http://phoenixalchemy.net

@phoenixalchemy

info@phoenixalchemy.net

Dancing in the Shadows:
A Healer's Perspective on Mental Health Crisis

By Olivia Kachman

Sunshine filtered through the curtains, casting shadows of birds chirping on a beautiful Saturday morning in June. My loving partner held my hand, his eyes filled with compassion and worry, as I lay beside him trembling and tearful in bed. My typical day for three weeks had been opening my eyes in the morning, feeling the rush of adrenaline that had me vomiting within minutes, and making it to the couch to focus on my breathing for hours, to self-regulate. I had no energy or will to engage in basic self-care, and my body had begun to deteriorate with my loss of appetite and dehydration. I was utterly exhausted, and yet could not sleep. Despite being seen as a healer and a helper in my community, I felt helpless in preventing the downward spiral I was experiencing, so I asked my partner to drive me to the nearest hospital emergency room.

The hours passed as we waited to see an emergency room doctor at the downtown hospital. My partner held me as I silently reflected on how my normally positive and optimistic frame of mind had become poisoned by racing thoughts of fear, self-doubt, hopelessness, and despair. It was as though a switch flicked off in my brain and I found myself in a self-destructive nightmare. My mind was a movie with images of a thousand ways I could end my life: jumping off the High Level Bridge, hanging myself, lunging in front of traffic, slitting my throat. It was hard to observe these relentless scenarios and not to get sucked into the darkness of despair. After I admitted to suicidal ideation, and two near attempts to suicide, the emergency room doctor immediately issued a Form 1 certification, which would prevent me from leaving the hospital for my own safety.

Three days waiting on an uncomfortable gurney in the ER, listening to electronic beeps and alarms, wailing or angry patients, clinical interviews, staff debriefs at shift changes, and the surveillance of security guards was unnerving. I remember how the green-tinted florescent lights glared at me as I was escorted down the empty, tiled hallway of the psychiatric ward upon my 11:00 p.m. arrival. The night shift psych nurse greeted me with a well-practiced compassionate smile. She led me into a white-walled room for "a few more questions" based on my admittance forms.

One series of questions really stood out, and I knew it was a trap: "Do you think you have any superpowers?" "No." "Do you hear voices in your head?" "No." Do you see things that are not real?" "No, of course not." I flatly lied to her, knowing that truthful answers would not serve me here. "Is that all?" I asked impatiently. "Can I just go to sleep now?" I said, hoping for a more comfortable bed and a night of uninterrupted sleep for the first time in weeks. I was rewarded with a standard hospital gown, a sleeping pill, and a bed that smelled of piss and sanitizer in a room with three other sedated women. "I will give you your orientation in the morning," the nurse said over her shoulder as she sharply drew the curtain closed. I sobbed myself to sleep that night, curled up in the fetal position.

The fluorescent lights flashed on promptly at 7:30 a.m. My orientation day in the psych ward had officially begun. Every detail of the unit was sterile, just as the food was bland. We were stripped of our possessions and the clothes we arrived in. We were under constant surveillance by nurses, psychiatrists, security guards, and video cameras. We had to earn our freedoms over time, which was such an institutionalized way of treating people who were suffering mentally. Essentially, we were in holding cells, killing time rather than harming ourselves or others, waiting for the effects of the medication cocktail to kick in. If we were lucky, the side effects would not cause us to feel worse, and if so, there was a pill for that too! To be clear, I am not against medication as an intervention; finding the right drug *saved my life*. I was just baffled at how highly educated hospital psychiatrists and pharmacists I talked to, admitted to having no clue which medication would successfully stabilize each patient's unique constitution. Some of the nurses and doctors were compassionate in their care, and some you could tell had their own stigma towards mental health. I also learned that, within the hospital, those who served in the realm of mental health were stigmatized by other doctors and nurses. Stigma affected everyone.

Ironically, if any one of those health care professionals had met me prior to my crisis in 2015, they would have known a heart-led woman who was following her soul's calling to empower people to reclaim their personal well-being. I have supported people in the transformation of their lives through energy work and shamanic journeys designed to heal the root cause of a trauma or issue. I also facilitate Kundalini Dance ™ as ceremonial movement medicine for the mind, body, and spirit. These modalities helped me to change my life from the inside out, and I felt inspired to guide others in doing the same.

As a woman on a spiritual journey, awakening her ancestral gifts, I knew that I had been developing "superpowers," which are not well known by modern psychiatry and are often misdiagnosed as psychosis or schizophrenia. I had come to realize that I was an intuitive empath with the abilities of clairvoyance (clearly seeing light, images, or symbols in the mind's eye), clairaudience (inner hearing from spiritual realms), clairsentience (the ability to feel and sense Spirit), and claircognizance (the ability to know, download information, or receive ideas and guidance). It had become my new normal to receive images or listen to the voices of my ancestors and spirit guides.

As a Transformational Guide in my business *Phoenix Alchemy*, I was the one helping others to navigate the shadows of stuck emotions, mental health crisis, childhood trauma, self-imposed limitations, or difficult life transitions. Yet here I was, trapped in the prison of my own mind, poisoned by negative thoughts. I felt so ashamed that despite having so many tools in my self-help toolkit, I could not access them in a suicidal or anxious state. I was about as far away from acceptance and love for myself as I could be; I judged myself harshly and felt like a fraud. While I isolated myself, not wanting to be seen in such a state, the people I generally trusted to reach out to, distanced themselves; either because of the stigma associated with mental illness, or because they did not know how to support someone who was struggling with these issues. Most of them just wanted the old version of Olivia to return, so when she didn't, they disappeared, and I retreated into self-isolation.

MENTAL HEALTH RECOVERY REQUIRES WHOLE HUMAN HEALING

In my view, a mental health crisis is a full systemic crisis of our physical, emotional, mental, and spiritual bodies.

There are layers and levels to our human experience, that energetically extend outwards from our physical body make up what is called an aura. The illustration below provides an easy way to visualize this concept. The different 'bodies' are stacked in connecting nested layers, starting with the physical and etheric bodies, then progressively moving out to the emotional body, the mental body, the astral body, and finally, the levels on the spiritual plane.

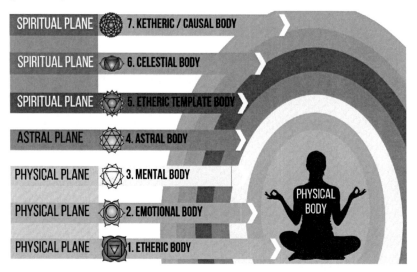

Source: https://www.psychicstudent.com/chakra-colours-and-meanings/

In my observation, a mental health crisis is initiated either from a spiritual disconnection filtering down through the energy layers into the physical body, or from a trauma in the physical-emotional body that affects each adjacent layer up to the spiritual body. Either way, when our aura is compromised, so is our immunity, our resilience, and our ability to filter out negative thought forms and influences, or even spiritual interference. What concerns me is that these elements of whole human health were hardly mentioned or even addressed in the health care system.

PHYSICAL BODY

Embodiment (In-Body-Meant) is about pure presence in your body, in this moment, right now. The past and future do not exist, so once we can anchor in the present, we can come back to ourselves and our lives; we can allow for a course correction. Deep healing, forgiveness, self-love, and the return of trust and faith all follow. For many, re-connecting to the physical body is a key. It is important for those around you to continually remind you that you are safe in your body and in this moment.

It would have been helpful for my own recovery to know about:

- Essential nutritional supplements and diet modifications that support mental health based on the proven gut-brain connection
- Techniques for calming the nervous system from the sympathetic (cortisol and adrenaline fight or flight responses) to the parasympathetic (relaxed and resting state)

- How unprocessed emotions get locked in the physical body and how to remedy that
- How to become 'embodied' again if we had dissociated from our physical bodies

With the intense anxiety I experienced, I became dissociated from my body. It gave me the sensation of being disconnected from the waist down, which sometimes felt like paralysis as my body went into "freeze" mode.   It felt like I had no legs, let alone a solid foundation to stand on.   It was incredibly frustrating for me because many of my wellness strategies are kinesthetic: movement-based like dance, yoga, swimming, and walking. Not being able to engage in these activities only added to my depressed state.

Through my experience I came to realize that in order to begin healing, it is critical for people to feel safe, fully embodied, and present in their physical bodies, and able to notice the sensations of temperature, tension, pain, comfort, and relaxation.   Our physical bodies are incredibly intelligent systems that send us messages all the time, if we tune in and listen. One way I avoided a lot of guesswork in choosing a medication, was by applying the technique of muscle testing, which essentially taps into my body's own intelligence and shows what drug or combination of drugs would be compatible with my body chemistry.

My mental health did not begin to improve until I found ways to be in my body and to become more present and accepting of where I was in the moment. Some things that helped me become more embodied included:

- Acknowledging my body through self-massage, patting myself into my body, stretching, and listening to what my body sensations were trying to communicate
- Using a Mantra: "I am allowed to feel in my body. I am allowed to feel safe in my body. This body belongs to me."
- Using heavy or weighted blankets when lying down resting helped me feel safe
- Stomping my feet, jumping up and down, shaking out all of my limbs for a few minutes
- Eventually returning to activities that had cardio and dynamic lower body exercises:
    - dance, yoga, squats and lunges, power walks, skipping rope, aerobics
    - taking up martial arts, kickboxing, and court sports

EMOTIONAL BODY

The losses and traumas that have affected the emotional landscape of an individual are not entirely validated or addressed by hospital staff or some mental health therapists but are left to unaffordable sessions with psychologists and counsellors. Depression, for example, can been described as the repression of emotion or, in contrast, an emotional overload from an accumulation of past events that leads to an experience of numbness, a lack of energy, vitality, and enjoyment of daily life. Anxiety, in contrast, is anchored in fear of the future and the person's ability to survive, which affects the nervous system with a primal response.

People need to feel that their emotions are validated. They need to have a safe space where they are encouraged to feel their grief and sadness, anger, and frustration, as well as the wounded trinity of abandonment, rejection, and betrayal that has accumulated. Where are these safe spaces where people can go to emotionally release these emotions without judgment? While in the psych ward, I knew with certainty that if I accessed and released my emotions below the layer of numbness, I would be put in an isolation room in the hospital! I can confidently say that we need to access our strong emotions like anger and grief, while being witnessed by someone who is supporting us to find our way through our labyrinth of hurt.

Here are some of the techniques I used to help me heal my emotional body:

- Emotional Freedom Technique (EFT) in a group therapy session
- Reactivating an emotion and offering it to the Earth or to Spirit in deep surrender
- Crying it out, roaring, stomping, cathartic yelling, amplifying the emotion until it is done
- Shadow Work® Process co-created by Cliff Barry and Mary Ellen Whalen
- Any form of dance or exercise that helps move emotion through the physical body

CASE STUDY: EMOTIONAL RELEASE IN KUNDALINI DANCE™

Dance is considered to be medicine in many communities and cultures around the world; it is the union of the physical, the emotional, and the spiritual; it goes beyond the thinking mind. Kundalini Dance is a ceremony where dancers are grounded, embodied, and connected to Spirit while exploring intuitive free movement. As a facilitator, I also led a portion of the class through a group session of emotional release. Imagine twenty-five people in a safe and confidential space, allowing whatever emotion comes up to erupt to the surface for acknowledgement and full expression for up to ten minutes. Imagine each person tuning in to their body sensations, signals, and emotions, allowing expression rather than repression! This act in itself changes lives. Not only is it cathartic, but I truly believe that we are not meant to be isolated in the experience of our emotions. We are meant to feel and be witnessed by others, unlike what we have been told. We are meant to let our emotions flow in order to let them go.

MENTAL BODY

I have personally discovered that thought patterns and behaviors really should be addressed after the nervous system has been stabilized (physical body), life force energy has been cultivated again after a period of rest (etheric body), and strong emotions have been processed (emotional body) to the extent that they are not overtaking the mind's ability to access reason, logic, and some level of objectivity. A suicidal, depressed, or anxious person creates very deep ruts in their brains, making neural connections that are based on self-hatred, negative bias, or fear-based reactions. Depending on how long they have ruminated in these directions, it takes time, constant self-awareness, and a whole lot of practice to create new positive, loving, and self-honoring neural pathways in the brain. Once they are more physically and emotionally settled, many people make the mistake of going back to work and familiar life routines without first spending enough time working on their thoughts, beliefs, word choice, and biases.

Here are some of the techniques that I have used to revive my mental body:

- Belief Re-patterning®, developed by Suze Casey, which involves a simple seven step process
- Mindfulness: to return to the present moment and sit with my thoughts
- Cognitive Behavioral Therapy (CBT) groups or one-on-one sessions
- Hypnotherapy or shamanic healing, to remove false beliefs or rewrite old contracts in the subconscious mind to be life-affirming
- Daily gratitude practice, before going to sleep, to reflect on the good in my day

SPIRITUAL BODY

You may resonate with the idea that you are "a spiritual being having a human experience" rather than a "human being having a spiritual experience." Either way, spirituality is universal among all cultures, regardless of religion. Every human being has a spiritual nature; awakening to that fact can be either subtle or dramatic. For people who do not relate to their spirit, it could be the missing link to their full sense of wellness.

Personally, my spiritual awakening has really accelerated since my early thirties and has become a central part of my life. My sense of connection to my higher self, spirit guides, animal guides, ancestors, spiritual allies, Creator and all of creation, brings me a sense of comfort and support. As I plummeted into a deep depression, it felt like there was a complete disconnection and separation from Spirit; an experience commonly referred to as the "dark nights of the soul." My sense of being alone, separate, and consumed by the void, felt like spiritual torture. It was a challenging test of my hope and faith that the realm of Spirit would not abandon me; that it would always be in me and around me, no matter what my mind told me.

Key rituals for connecting to one's Spirit might include:

- Praying or meditating
- Singing, toning, reciting mantras or affirmations
- Playing classical music or healing frequencies
- Reading scripture or inspiring texts
- Creating your own ritual or ceremony for any occasion
- Walking with complete presence in nature with awe
- Observing the synchronicities in your life with gratitude
- Accessing "the zone" in sport, writing, music, dance, or art

SHAMANIC HEALING AS WHOLE PERSON HEALTH CARE

Shamanism is one of the most ancient modalities of medicine in the world and exists across all cultures. I have developed a deep appreciation for shamanic healing because of how fluidly and gently it addresses the interconnection of the physical, emotional, mental, and spiritual aspects of a human being. Miraculous shifts in whole person healing and perception occur in ways that modern psychiatry does not recognize, but quantum physics is beginning to provide an explanation for.

A common practice of a shamanic practitioner is tracking the root cause of a wounded psyche in the mental body, which leads to "time travelling" the person's physical body to the first moment in time-space where that trauma became embedded. Unlike talk therapy, shamanic healing allows for a gentle energetic release where none of the experience is relived or even discussed; which can be retraumatizing. The first law of thermodynamics states that energy is neither created nor destroyed, only transformed from one form to another. Energy in motion is defined by many holistic practitioners as emotion; any stuck or hardened energy resulting from a traumatic event requires emotional transmutation. The wounded psyche of false beliefs can then be reprogrammed by guiding the person into a trance state where they can access their subconscious, delete what is false, and insert what feels empowering.

Looking through the shamanic lens of reality, ongoing patterns are often ancestral and are recorded in our DNA. Whether these ancestral patterns show up as mental health challenges and addiction, fears and phobias, or intergenerational trauma, it is possible for us to address them this lifetime and not pass them forward. I have heard the expression that "we are the ones our ancestors prayed for," and I think it applies here in the sense that by finding the strength and courage within ourselves to resolve these inherited or acquired issues in the present, we are also resolving them in the past. Similarly, the aboriginal expression,

"For all my Relations," recognizes the power of our personal healing on seven generations into the past and into the future.

Wouldn't it be amazing if shamanic practitioners who have this knowledge could work alongside health care professionals? They could help patients address mental health challenges and addictions, as well as disease and traumas, from a different angle.

CASE STUDY: TRACKING THE ROOT CAUSE OF A MENTAL HEALTH ISSUE

I was able to help a woman I spent time with, the night before she was discharged from the hospital. She related to me that she had been plagued by extreme anxiety her entire life and could not remember when it had started, but that she "could hardly breathe." I was beginning to feel more embodied at this stage of my hospital stay and I took a moment to tune into her. I muscle tested for her to find out how old she was when she first couldn't breathe. The event occurred when she was about one year old, and the anxiety had really taken root in her psyche by the age of two and half.

She immediately burst into tears; I just sat and let her cry. She recalled her parents telling her how she had found her way into the pasture as a toddler and had been kicked in the chest by a horse. She had gone flying through the air. No one was watching her at the time. As an adult, she had always felt a sense of abandonment. Where were the people who loved her? Unable to breathe and unconscious, she had been driven to the hospital; everyone on board was panicking, afraid that she would die.

Panic attacks where she could hardly breathe and felt like she was dying, had been her experience for 40 years. She was able to connect the dots in her conscious awareness with that simple tracking technique; it was enough to give her hope. The next day she awoke from the deepest sleep she had had in weeks. She had a smile on her face, hope in her heart, and was actually looking forward to going home and addressing the root cause of her anxiety and panic attacks through therapy.

CASE STUDY: MY EXPERIENCE OF HEALING WITH SHADOW WORK

The crackle of the wood stove fire brought a comfort to the womb-like sacred space of the yurt where I sat cross-legged with others who had chosen to face their shadows with courage. Two highly skilled facilitators trained in Shadow Work- a combination of psychotherapy and archetypal healing- gave us the opportunity, one by one, to face our personal demons, self-imposed limitations, and deepest fears.

It was my turn to rise and face my own shadow- the voice telling me to kill myself; that I was worthless and had no place in this world. I had been hearing this voice on and off for a year and a half since leaving the hospital, and it was growing louder and more insistent. Something in me was drawn to this circle process, despite feeling suicidal and wanting to give up.

I was given the chance to play out the voices in my head between my Inner Judge and my Inner Warrior, but symbolically, in front of my eyes. Through the depths of repressed rage, I ignited my Inner Warrior again to fight for my Life. By activating my Inner Warrior archetype that I thought was long gone, I defeated my Inner Judge and claimed my worth. I proclaimed that I had a place in this world and belonged here! This strong voice came from deep inside of me. I felt a light touch in every cell of my body as I opened to this truth that had been blotted out by darkness. I was alive and I did belong! I had things to do that were important! I needed to find my way back to life again.

The circle celebrated this personal victory with a dance and a group hug. This process helped me to access my willpower and gain momentum. Slowly but surely, I began to spiral upwards out of depression. Accessing my raging Inner Warrior in the safe and sacred space of that yurt, while being witnessed and supported by others, was a crucial experience in my own healing journey.

FINAL REFLECTION

Much of what I've shared here has detailed my first experience with what has been diagnosed as Major Depressive Disorder with acute anxiety. I chalked up my experience to coming off epilepsy medications (my doctors hadn't told me that they had mood stabilizers in them), compassion fatigue from an intense job in social work while operating my soul-calling of shamanic healing on the side, and a generalized existential crisis. I truly thought that I would never experience that level of darkness again, but, looking back now, I am not sure if I ever entirely came through my original depression. My full recovery was tossed aside when I was once again confronted with high stress situations, such as navigating my dad's cancer treatments and dealing with his death, the dissolution of our family acreage, moving my mother to the city, and the end of my partnership of nearly seven years. Little did I know that major depression has an eighty percent recurrence rate.

Just as I was leading this book project into the structural editing phase, I experienced my second major bout of suicidal depression and anxiety. I was voluntarily hospitalized for two months. Since then, the shame has been intense, despite my desire to speak out and become an advocate for mental health. I could hardly tell my co-authors. Seeing this book through to completion has become one reason for me to practice being courageous and to keep going in the midst of intense darkness. I am in the initial steps of recovery as I write this, still taking things one day at a time; struggling, but feeling more clear-minded. The constant barrage of suicidal thoughts is now quiet, and I can begin the process of self-healing, receiving therapy, and obtaining the support I need.

From light to shadows and from shadows to light, I am facing what it means to be a phoenix as I face challenges in my own mental health. I am discovering that we are not meant to heal on our own. I have come to realize that there are big gaps in how our current health care approaches mental health, and I would like to inspire change. I am finding my voice to be an advocate for mental health, despite feeling the stigma and facing my own sense of shame and self-stigma. I am learning how to love and accept myself: in darkness, in light, and in every shade of grey.

Despite all of the challenges I have faced, I am slowly but surely rising again, "For all my Relations."

Personal Insights: From Shadows to Light

- It is important to be proactive and gather a health care team that includes western medical doctors and holistic practitioners *before* you have a health crisis, so you have the support of people you trust and who know your history.

- True empathy is a lifesaver, as it is important to know that you are not alone. Often family members, friends, colleagues, and health care professionals will not be able to empathize with you unless they have personally experienced similar mental health challenges.

- In-person peer support or therapy groups, as well as online groups and crisis lines are essential social support networks.

- All healthcare professionals, caregivers, social service professionals, holistic practitioners, first responders, crisis line operators and veterans need access to better support systems in place for compassion fatigue, trauma and PTSD recovery in their workplaces. These groups are at risk for developing mental health issues and must feel safe and supported in a 'no shame' workplace where people look out for one another.

- I would like to see the opening of a center that addresses the physical, emotional, mental, and spiritual bodies. I have written down the physical blueprint of this building concept, and I envision that someday centers like this will be available all over the world as places for community healing. Will you help me to make this real?

Conclusion

I did not know what true courage was until embarking on this mission to gather people to talk about their mental health journeys and their paths to recovery. In these pages, we have endeavored to face our own traumas and triggers bravely; vulnerably recounting our personal experiences to voice solidarity with those of you facing challenges in your own mental health. For nearly half the authors, this book marks their first time publishing their personal stories, and we had no concept of how much self-doubt, fear, shame, and personal challenges we would have to overcome to keep writing. It is our hope that you saw your own courage and resilience reflected in the pages of this compilation.

As discussed in the Introduction, anyone who has first-hand experience with mental health challenges is an Initiate, and I am convinced that Initiates should lead the conversation and reform around mental health. In interviewing potential co-authors for this book, I was taken aback by how many had experienced significant traumas, stigma, and shame. It seems apparent that trauma can be a primary root cause of mental health and addiction challenges, beyond factors like genetics, epigenetics, or even our diets and stress. It begs the question: who are the service providers within our health care system treating the root cause of trauma effectively with a whole human approach?

Mental health recovery is a multi-faceted subject that requires a nuanced approach to effectively address. The power of this compilation, then, lies in the pieces of the puzzle offered by each co-author's contribution to the dialogue around the physical and emotional bodies, mind, and spirit in approaching mental health recovery. For instance, it is important to consider body-based somatic and energy healing to track the root cause of trauma in the body and release it. It is clear that approaches that address intergenerational family trauma are just as critical as those that address the personal traumas of our current lifetime. In addition, our brains physiologically change with the experience of trauma or mental health decline. As a result, optimal nutrition plays as critical a role in recovery, as does the necessary transformation of negative thoughts, wounded beliefs, and shame. It was our intent to increase awareness of the spectrum of alternative resources available to address mental health challenges, which complement the use of conventional interventions, such as medication or group therapy.

Just as the friends and family of a diagnosed diabetic should be educated about the signs, symptoms, and helpful interventions associated with the diagnosis, it is important that people become informed about mental health in the same way. Peer support and an educated public are absolutely critical at a grassroots level. You may even have acknowledged ways in which you may have contributed to spreading the stigma about mental health, and how you can begin to change that.

We all have a role to play in creating a society that is more compassionate, empathetic, and socially inclusive. Together, we can dismantle the social stigma that keeps mental health challenges in the shadows.

Afterword

By Deeanne Riendeau of Your Holistic Earth

Our western medical system was built to address acute illness and injury. It was an immediate need and an extremely valuable solution for the time in which it was created. However, the pressures that currently face our medical system mean that something has to change.

From Shadows to Light offers a glorious response to an all-too-common problem in our communities: how can we nurture and improve the health of our whole beings rather than just one part of us at a time? The authors of this compilation have bravely shared their own struggles to convey that you are not alone, and you are capable of healing yourself with support. They have distilled their decades of professional experience down to actionable steps to remind us that there is hope. And they have pointed the reader, again and again, to the vast, yet often invisible, array of resources available to fulfill whole-person wellness.

For many of you, Your Holistic Earth (yourholisticearth.ca) could be one step on your journey to living a more holistic lifestyle, depending less on conventional medicine and more on nature's own cures. For others, the journey has already begun, and you seek information and resources to incorporate additional holistic therapies into your daily regimen and practice.

At Your Holistic Earth, our goal is to be the bridge that connects you to the local and national experts in the field of holistic medicine. Through our community, you will find support and resources to help you learn more about living healthier and feeling better every day. We have partnered with the best practitioners in the industry to make it easy for you to step into a more holistic lifestyle, supported by experts who care.

It is my belief that our ability to help one another to heal begins by healing ourselves. It starts with you.

Deeanne Riendeau
President & Founder
https://yourholisticearth.ca/

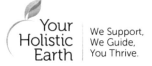

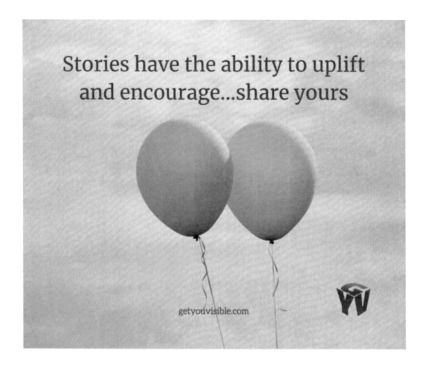

Stories have the ability to uplift and encourage...share yours

getyouvisible.com

Do You Dream of Being a Published Author?

The best part of what I do is bringing people together to write, share, and inspire those that may feel alone or in need of healing. Your story could help to heal others.

My team will guide you through the writing process, so your idea can become a reality to be shared on worldwide distribution channels.

A book has been referenced as an authority piece for centuries and is known to be one of the best ways to gain instant credibility and visibility with clients in the online and offline space.

If you have a story to share and want to become a published author or co-author in a collaborative, then let's talk. Here's to your story and someone waiting to read it.

Book your complimentary call with me.
www.getyouvisible.com

Join us:
https://www.facebook.com/groups/getyouvisiblecommunity

See you on the other side.

Heather Andrews
CEO, Get You Visible